RESEARCHING LANGUAGE AND HEALTH

Researching Language and Health explores key topics in illness and healthcare contexts through multiple linguistic lenses.

This book highlights key themes, guides readers through the design stages of research and the ethical considerations specific to linguistic health research, and brings methods and methodologies to life by demonstrating how these can be applied to specific issues in context. Covering a wide range of health conditions, healthcare contexts, and data types, with an emphasis on those most accessible to students and new researchers, the authors foreground the 'so what?' of research and the impact that linguistic studies can have.

Both a guide to key elements of the research process and a holistic view of research projects that have been successful, insightful, and impactful in different contexts, this is an essential text for advanced students and researchers in healthcare communication and applied linguistics.

Zsófia Demjén is Associate Professor of Applied Linguistics at University College London. Her main research interests are language and discourses around illness, with recent projects focusing on depression, psychosis, cancer, and vaccinations. She uses a range of analytical tools including discourse, metaphor, narrative, and corpus analysis.

Sarah Atkins is Teaching and Research Fellow at Aston University with research interests in language and communication in professional contexts. She has worked on a number of projects within healthcare and health education, with a focus on the practical relevance of findings for practitioners.

Elena Semino is Professor of Linguistics and Verbal Art in the Department of Linguistics and English Language at Lancaster University, and Director of the ESRC Centre for Corpus Approaches to Social Science. She specializes in health communication, medical humanities, corpus linguistics, stylistics, narratology and metaphor theory and analysis.

RESEARCHING LANGUAGE AND HEALTH

A Student Guide

Zsófia Demjén
Sarah Atkins
Elena Semino

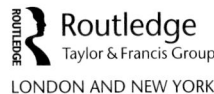

Routledge
Taylor & Francis Group
LONDON AND NEW YORK

Designed cover image: © Getty Images | peepo

First published 2024
by Routledge
4 Park Square, Milton Park, Abingdon, Oxon OX14 4RN

and by Routledge
605 Third Avenue, New York, NY 10158

Routledge is an imprint of the Taylor & Francis Group, an informa business

British Library Cataloguing-in-Publication Data
A catalogue record for this book is available from the British Library

ISBN: 978-0-367-89669-0 (hbk)
ISBN: 978-0-367-89668-3 (pbk)
ISBN: 978-1-003-02041-7 (ebk)

DOI: 10.4324/9781003020417

Typeset in Bembo
by Deanta Global Publishing Services, Chennai, India

CONTENTS

ACKNOWLEDGEMENTS

Many have contributed to the making of this book, including all the researchers whose work we feature throughout and we thank them for their work. A few additional thanks are also in order:

We would like to thank Chris West, Kate Miller, Gill Ereaut, Dr Emmet Ó Briain, and Kevin McLean for their permission to draw on their LinkedIn discussions in Chapter 4. We would also like to thank Dr Kitty Li for helping us with the early research for parts of the book. Thank you to Dr Kevin Harvey for his discussion of the study featured in Chapter 9 and for his permission to use it in the book. We are grateful to Professor Celia Roberts and Professor Kamila Hawthorne for their insightful comments on the research partnership discussed in Chapter 12. We are also enormously grateful to the Principal Investigator of the Schwartz Rounds project, Dr Laura Thompson, for permission to use the case study in Chapter 13 of this book. Finally, we would like to thank our editor, Louisa Semlyen, and editorial assistants Talitha Duncan-Todd, and Eleni Steck for their encouragement and patience throughout the writing process.

We greatly appreciate the funding that our various projects have received. These projects have provided us with much of the experience we are able to share here. Specifically: The Metaphor in End-of-Life Care project featured in Chapter 8 was funded by the UK's Economic and Social Research Council (grant number: ES/J007927/1). The Questioning Vaccination Discourse project featured in Chapters 8 and 11 was funded by the Economic and Social Research Council, part of UK Research and Innovation (ES/V000926/1, 2021–2024). The project on health professionals' communication through role-play featured in Chapter 12 was funded by a Knowledge Transfer Partnership award (KTP008346, 2011–2013) and by an Economic and Social Research Council 'Future Research Leaders' grant at the University of Nottingham (ES/K00865X/1, 2013–2016). The project on Schwartz Rounds discussed in Chapter 13 was funded by a Wellcome Trust Institutional Strategic Support Fund at Birkbeck, University of London.

We have received permission to reproduce the following:

Chapter 4, Example 4.1: From Mulderrig, J. (2017) Reframing obesity: a critical discourse analysis of the UK's first social marketing campaign, *Critical Policy Studies*, 11:4, 455–76. Reprinted with permission from Taylor & Francis via Copyright Clearance Center.

Chapter 4, Figure 4.6: From Oyebode, O., Unuabonah, F. O. (2013) Coping with HIV/AIDS: A multimodal discourse analysis of selected HIV/AIDS posters in south-western Nigeria. *Discourse and Society*, 24(6): 810–27. Reprinted by Permission of SAGE Publications

Chapter 5, Figure 1: From Elizabeth Swados, *My Depression: A Picture Book*. Copyright ©2005 by Elizabeth Swados. Reprinted with the permission of The Permissions Company, LLC on behalf of Seven Stories Press, sevenstories.com.

Chapter 5, Figure 2: From Rachel Ball, *The Inflatable Woman*. Copyright ©2015 by Rachel Ball. Reprinted with the permission of the author.

Chapter 6, Example 6.6: From Swinglehurst, D. (2015) How linguistic ethnography may enhance our understanding of electronic patient records in health care settings. In J. Snell, S. Shaw, & F. Copland (Eds.), Linguistic Ethnography (pp. 90–109). Basingstoke: Palgrave Macmillan. Reprinted with permission from Elsevier via Copyright Clearance Center.

Chapter 8, Examples 8.17–8.20: From Stommel, W. and Koole, T. (2010) The online support group as a community: A micro-analysis of the interaction with a new member. *Discourse Studies*, 12(3), 357–8. Reprinted by Permission of SAGE Publications.

Chapter 8, Figure 8.1: From Koteyko, N., & Hunt, D. (2016). Performing health identities on social media: An online observation of Facebook profiles. Discourse, Context & Media, 12, 59–67. Reprinted with permission from Elsevier via Copyright Clearance Center.

Chapter 9, Figures 9.1–9.3: From Harvey, K. (2013). Medicalisation, pharmaceutical promotion, and the Internet: a critical multimodal discourse analysis of hair loss websites. *Social Semiotics*, 23(5): 691–714. Reprinted with permission from Routledge.

Chapter 4, Figures 4.7 and 4.8: we contacted Jive Media for permission to reprint these images on several occasions between May and December 2022. After an initial positive response, our emails went unanswered. The images are reproduced under a CC-BY-NC-ND licence, with credit to Jive Media and the CDC.

PART I
Planning your research

1

INTRODUCTION TO *RESEARCHING LANGUAGE AND HEALTH*

1.1 Introduction

Illness and health are among the most central and universal human concerns. As we write this book, most countries in the world are still grappling with the effects of a global pandemic; we all get ill and we all need to be well to lead the lives we want to lead. Language is also universally human and we use it to express and mediate most aspects of illness and healthcare. This book, therefore, is dedicated to the fascinating intersection of language and health, introducing how we can use the former to understand the latter. We intend the book as a point of reference and orientation in a vast field, making accessible an area that can sometimes seem as daunting as it is important. We showcase the kinds of topics and data that could be explored, demonstrate many reasons why language in the context of health is important to study, and introduce our readers to tools, methods, and approaches that will enable them to design and carry out studies of language use (both verbal and non-verbal) in healthcare contexts.

Health is conceived broadly in this book to include any human illness or condition, the care that one might give or receive, wellness and wellbeing, the behaviours intended to maintain it, and anything that might jeopardize it. Language of, around, or about this broad conception of health, whether in public or more private spaces, can take a dizzying array of forms well beyond traditional doctor–patient interactions in a clinic. It can include anything from water safety information to adverts for various forms of physical enhancement; from things people read before seeing their clinicians, to how surgeons gesture in the operating theatre; from media reports about novel pathogens and public service announcements, to films and (graphic) novels featuring characters with different conditions, and the conversations (and silences) people have about health or such texts, among many others. Examples 1–5 in this chapter present

DOI: 10.4324/9781003020417-2

a taster of the range of data we cover in this book. All language around health is worthy of study and can lead to different socially and individually relevant insights.

Looking in detail at the language used when doctors talk to patients, as in Example 1.1, can lead to insights about the impact that small, seemingly insignificant words such as 'any' can have on how an interaction unfolds. Research has shown that in questions and invites 'any' tends to elicit a 'no' response more often than a 'yes' (Heritage et al., 2007). In a context like Example 1.1, where the doctor is quickly running through a history, such questions work well.

EXAMPLE 1.1   From Boyd & Heritage, 2006, discussed in Chapter 6

```
 1   Doctor:  -> An' do you have any other medical problems?
 2   Patient:    Uh: no.
 3                  (7.0)
 4   Doctor:     No heart disease,
 5   Patient:    #Hah:.# ((cough))
 6   Patient:    No.
 7                  (1.3)
 8   Doctor:  -> Any lung disease as far as you know:,
 9   Patient:    No.
10                  (.)
11   Patient:    Not that I know of.
12                  (.)
13   Doctor:  -> Any diabetes,
14   Patient:    No.
15   Doctor:  -> Have you ever had (uh) surgery?
16                  (0.5)
17   Patient:    I've had four surgeries on my left knee:.
```

However, if a doctor is asking a patient about additional concerns as in, 'Is there anything else you'd like to discuss today?', *any*-questions make it less likely that the patient will feel able to raise them. Such insights can be used to inform the training of healthcare professionals.

Exploring ways in which one particular behaviour, for instance breastfeeding in Example 1.2, is represented in contrast with another behaviour (e.g. bottle feeding in Example 1.3) can reveal underlying interests, aims, and assumptions of message producers (Brookes et al., 2016). If you contrast the titles and subtitles of the two leaflets in Example 1.2 and Example 1.3, breastfeeding is linked explicitly to 'the best start', which implies that any other feeding choice is inferior. Similarly, while the subtitle of this leaflet describes the contents in relatively neutral terms as 'important information', the contents of the bottle feeding leaflet are described in more negatively valenced terms as 'to minimize the risks'.

EXAMPLE 1.2   Front page of a Start 4 Life parenting leaflet on breastfeeding, discussed in Chapter 4

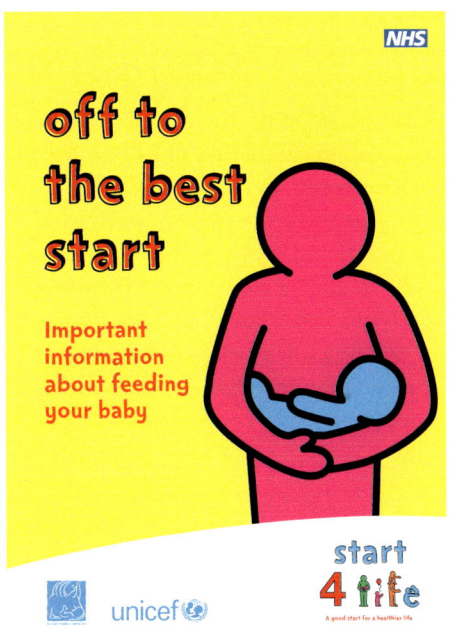

EXAMPLE 1.3   Front page of a Start 4 Life parenting leaflet on bottle feeding, discussed in Chapter 4

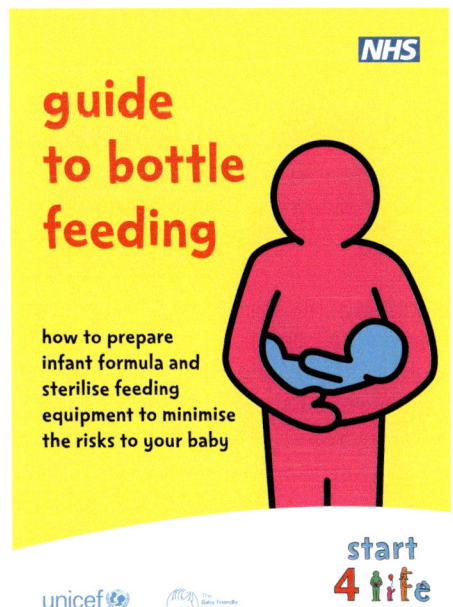

The message producers clearly position breastfeeding as the best and safest feeding option. But, as any parent will be able to attest, how one feeds one's child is not necessarily a question of free choice. Exploring these patterns allows us to question the, perhaps unintended, consequences that this kind of messaging might have for parents and their sense of self.

The depiction of different illnesses and conditions in fictional narratives such as novels (Example 1.4), films, and soap operas allows those without direct experience to immerse themselves in new worlds and empathize with perspectives they do not share. Analyzing such depictions can help us understand public attitudes to illnesses and conditions and think about the representations that exist and those that might be needed. Example 1.4 comes from Mark Haddon's *The Curious Incident of the Dog in the Night-Time* (2003), from a scene where Christopher, the narrator/protagonist, is being questioned by a policeman after being found holding the corpse of his next-door neighbour's dog, with a garden fork sticking out of its stomach (Semino, 2014).

> **EXAMPLE 1.4** From the published novel, The Curious Incident of a Dog in the Night-Time, discussed in Chapter 5
>
> The policeman squatted down beside me and said, 'Would you like to tell me what's going on here, young man?'
>   I sat up and said, 'The dog is dead.'
>   'I'd got that far,' he said.
>   I said, 'I think someone killed the dog.'
>   'How old are you?' he asked.
>   I replied, 'I am 15 years and 3 months and 2 days.'

Although it is never explicitly stated in the novel, readers have tended to conclude that Christopher's particular way of providing arguably too little information at certain points and too much at others represents some aspects of how someone with autism sees the world. Such fictional depictions can influence, reflect and reinforce public perceptions of different illnesses or conditions.

Harnessing quantitative corpus linguistic tools can enable us to see patterns in the language of media reports (Example 1.5), online forum contributions, or questions to healthcare professionals online that would otherwise be undetectable due to the sheer size and range of datasets. Example 1.5 for instance, is an excerpt from one of 627 articles on antimicrobial resistance (i.e. when bacteria, viruses, fungi, and parasites change over time and no longer respond to medicines) that appeared in the UK press between 2010 and 2015 (Collins et al., 2018). Similarly to other articles, Example 1.5 refers to antibiotics being 'used', but it is not explicit about who does the using (although from context it can be assumed that users are in farming and agriculture). Such representations – if they are prevalent – background the role that individuals play in the increase of anti-microbial resistance and can help explain why people may not understand how the health concern might affect them and what they can do to help resolve such wider issues.

EXAMPLE 1.5   A media report on antimicrobial resistance analyzed, discussed in Chapter 4

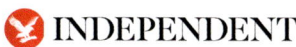 INDEPENDENT

NEWS   INDEPENDENT TV   CLIMATE   SPORT   VOICES   CULTURE   TRAVEL   INDY/LIFE

> The addition of antibiotics to feed to improve the growth rates of farm animals has been banned throughout the EU since 1 January 2006. Antibiotics are now only used under the prescription and care of a veterinary surgeon to combat and prevent bacterial infections which may cause animals to become sick, in the same way that humans use antibiotics.

Example 1.6 and Example 1.7 on the other hand come from a UK-based website called 'Teenage Health Freak', where adolescents are able to post about their health concerns and ask questions anonymously (Harvey, 2012). Here, corpus methods helped to show that there is a difference between teenagers saying 'i am depressed' and 'I have depression'.

EXAMPLE 1.6   From Harvey, 2012, discussed in Chapter 7

i am not happy with myself i am fat i get bullied and i am depressed

EXAMPLE 1.7   From Harvey, 2012, discussed in Chapter 7

I have depression, and it seems to be getting worse lately. i've been feeling horrible through most of the hols, and i still do even though im back at school.

'I am depressed' tended to be found in messages that ask for advice about the cause of negative feelings (e.g. getting bullied) rather than the negative feelings themselves. It seemed to capture an experience that is perhaps more transient. On the other hand, messages using 'I have depression' tended to ask for advice on how to handle the *consequences* of the feeling. This was a more clinical, potentially pathologizing view of negative emotions, which seemed to be perceived as a relatively stable.

As these examples demonstrate, health-related language can occur in many different settings, physical and virtual. It can be interactive, involving two or more parties in a/synchronous interactions, in-person, or mediated by some form of communication technology. It can be monologic and unidirectional, designed for narrow or broad audiences. It can, but need not, involve clinicians and other healthcare professionals. It can be institutional, carefully planned and designed, or free and spontaneous. It can be verbal and multimodal. Whatever contexts, settings, channels, modes, genres, or participants you pick, the language being used to communicate about and around illness and health will be revealing with regard to concerns, subjectivities, identities, relationships, ideologies, tensions, vulnerabilities, norms, values, systems, and resources involved. Taking a linguistic approach to health is different from the traditional 'biomedical model' of health. The latter focuses on biochemical explanations of ill health as the basis for treatment and intervention (Yuill et al., 2010). Linguistic analysis, of course, does not claim to treat disease, but it is nevertheless aligned with the 'biopsychosocial model' of health which recognizes that behaviours, thoughts and feelings may influence a physical state (McInerney, 2002). A linguistic approach to health recognizes that we can learn something about conditions, illnesses, and healthcare contexts from the ways in which they are talked and written about. This book introduces many tools to enable such learning.

1.2 Who is this book for?

This book is aimed at final year Undergraduates and Masters students working on their dissertations, PhD students preparing their research proposals and for more experienced scholars new to the domain. Novice researchers often have very similar questions at the start: what kind of data should I collect or generate? How much data do I need and where can I find it? How do I formulate research questions? What ethical concerns do I need to bear in mind? How can I analyze my data? These are exactly the kinds of questions that we address explicitly in specific chapters in Part I of the book, and in the preliminary considerations at the start of Part II chapters. More experienced researchers may want to start with specific types of insights that can be generated, or the kinds of tools that can be applied in a specific domain, and these are the subject of the central sections in Part II of the book. The case studies in Part III of the book collect practical lessons learned while researching language and health and will be relevant to all our audiences.

1.2.1 What this book does and does not cover

Research on communication around health and illness comes from many different disciplinary orientations, including philosophy, psychology, sociology, anthropology, and, of course, medicine. This book, however, is firmly rooted in Linguistics, and more specifically in discourse analytic approaches to language. 'Discourse' here refers to ways of representing (and therefore potentially thinking and reasoning about) different aspects of reality, and 'analytic' to the range of tools, techniques, and lenses that can be used to make sense of social life through the forms and functions of language as it is used in context. We cover a good number of these tools, techniques, and lenses including corpus linguistics, narrative analysis, pragmatics, digital ethnography, conversation analysis, interactional sociolinguistics, systemic functional linguistics, stylistics, metaphor analysis, critical discourse analysis, speech presentation, and multimodal social semiotics. None of these methods are unique to research on language and health, but the overviews we provide are rooted in this domain. We also refer our readers to broader, more detailed introductions to these methods for further information.

Doing applied linguistic analysis in the context of health is incredibly rewarding. There are so many different types of insights to be gained, from insights about the aetiology, phenomenology, diagnosis and treatment of different illnesses; how different linguistic phenomena manifest and are used in this specific context; how typical methodologies work and/or need to be adapted in this context; how communicative activities that make up healthcare work and/or need to be improved; to insights about sociocultural values, practices, and ideologies that underpin, influence, and are reinforced by how we experience and treat illness. That said, the discourse analytic approach is suitable for investigating certain aspects of health communication but not others. In this book we cover the following areas which can be studied using discourse analysis:

- Experience of illness, to reveal personal and social dimensions of what it means to be ill or work with people who are;
- Linguistic (re)presentation of self, others and illnesses or conditions in public messaging, mainstream media and peer-to-peer interactions, to lead to a better understanding of public perceptions of illness and healthcare and how we manage our selves when ill;
- Use of specific linguistic phenomena, such as metaphor or narratives, in healthcare contexts to understand the domain-specific roles they play;
- Role of different technologies in how people approach and express health concerns;
- Function and authenticity of communicative activities that are prominent in the training, assessment, and professional development of healthcare practitioners;
- Dyadic or group interactional behaviour in healthcare contexts to understand the development of communities and how different aspects of our identities, cultures and motivations come into play;
- Institutional and socio-political context of illness to understand pressures and influences that can bear down on micro-linguistic choices, but also how these choices connect with wider ideologies and might impact the most vulnerable in society.

As this list implies, there are also topics and approaches that we do not cover. We do not cover any experimental work on language and health, nor do we cover topics associated with Clinical Linguistics and Clinical Pragmatics, i.e. fields where language disorders are studied. For these topics readers can turn to excellent introductions already in existence (e.g. Cummings, 2008). We also do not provide detailed, step-by-step guidance on how to apply specific research methods. For such overviews, it is necessary to go beyond our book and we refer readers (both below and in subsequent chapters) to many fantastic resources that already exist.

Throughout this book, we have chosen to foreground topics, data types, methodologies, and concerns that will be most easily accessible to researchers and which, in our experience, tend to be of greatest interest to those beginning their explorations in this field. For example, we know that people are often interested in questions of identities and how these come into being in language and interaction. You will see that several chapters (e.g. Chapter 6 and 8) refer to Bucholtz and Hall's (2005) seminal sociolinguistic approach to identity, which sees it as emerging from discourse. The approach can and has been applied to different kinds of data, using different types of linguistic frameworks for analysis.

In thinking about the accessibility of topics and data types, we have considered both issues of access to research sites and participants and ethical implications and complexities that might arise. We have also prioritized topics that are possible to address in small-scale projects such as Undergraduate or Masters dissertations. In the research we describe, we foreground work that has been conducted on/in and published in English, but have made efforts to include work conducted in non-English-speaking settings. We make suggestions for what to bear in mind when researching other languages but writing in English, and we hope that the book will inspire research in other languages and contexts, using an even wider set of approaches.

1.3 Navigating this book

As indicated above, the structure of this book mirrors the thinking and learning process novice researchers tend to go through when they begin working towards an independent research project in language and health. Part I takes you through typical initial considerations to do with research questions, data selection, methodology, and ethics, when designing a project. Part II helps you narrow down your topic of focus, providing plenty of example studies addressing particular themes with different datasets and methods. Chapters in Part III then provide detailed case studies of how real projects have handled different challenges that can emerge in the research process. The parts, chapters, and sections of the book are extensively cross-referenced to enable both a cover-to-cover and a dip-in-and-out reading.

Following on from this introduction, Chapter 2 in Part I discusses the golden triangle of research questions, data, and research methods (Figure 1.1), showing how decisions about each of these will have an impact on the others. It explains how to formulate worthwhile and feasible research questions, how to identify and collect relevant data, and briefly outlines some principal methods suitable for different types of research questions and data. All sections are cross-referenced to other chapters and sections of the book where further details and examples can be found on how the advice we provide can be (and has been) put into practice.

Chapter 3 focuses in detail on ethical considerations and codes of conduct relevant for doing research on language and health, where sensitive data or vulnerable populations might be concerned. The ethical implications of any research project need to be part of the thinking and planning right from the start. We describe 'macro-ethical' principles of *respect* for participant autonomy, *beneficence*, *non-maleficence*, and *justice* in the way the research is conducted and provide accounts of some of the 'micro-ethical' difficulties linguistic researchers come up against when putting these principles into practice.

Rather than focusing on specific methods, chapters in Part II of the book immediately involve readers in the kinds of questions or issues that are of interest in the field, by focusing on types of data (e.g. literary representations of illness) combined with types of topics or concerns (e.g. the impact they can have on public perceptions of illness). The types of questions that can be asked and analytical approaches that can be taken emerge organically from these.

Chapters 4 and 5 cover widely published data types, which are in the public domain and therefore most easily accessible for novice researchers. Chapter 4 discusses questions that have been asked of and approaches taken to public health communications, including institutional public health campaigns and media reports. It explores issues around the (often implicit) linguistic allocation of agency and responsibility; the communication of risk and uncertainty; encouraging behaviour change; and considerations of different social, economic, and political contexts. Chapter 5 focuses on questions that can be asked of published novels and memoirs centred on personal experiences of different conditions and illnesses. These questions include the extent and ways in which such texts can improve our understanding of illness and how they might influence public perceptions of illnesses and the people who experience them.

Chapters 6 and 7 cover interactions offline and on, which are often seen as core types of language around health. Chapter 6 focuses on spoken, in-person interactions that take place in healthcare contexts. These are perhaps the least accessible types of data for student and novice researchers, but the chapter includes a number of suggestions on how to overcome this. Topics and issues that are highlighted as relevant for this kind of data include how relationships and power imbalances are negotiated between interlocutors, how identities can be constructed and the role that technology might play in such encounters. Chapter 7 then takes a look at virtual interactions between healthcare professionals and the public (sometimes patients), and public comments on healthcare services and health news. It focuses on subjects such as the challenges of providing expert health advice online, the importance of this kind of data for understanding what actually concerns different groups of people in relation to health, and understanding how people might perceive health threats and healthcare services and why.

Chapter 8 also centres on digital data and focuses on patients' lived experiences both in dialogic and monologic form. We have devoted two chapters to

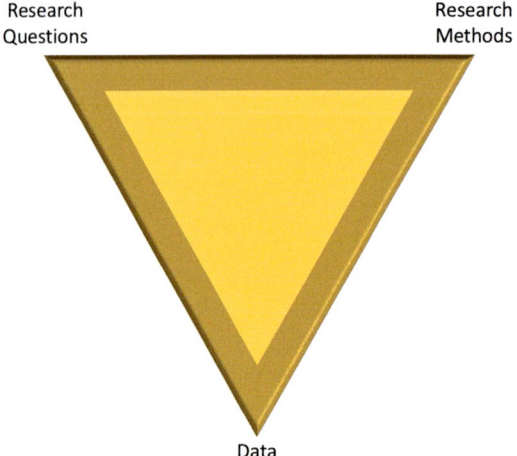

Research Questions

Research Methods

Data

FIGURE 1.1 The golden triangle of Research Questions, Methods, and Data

language that occurs in digital health contexts to reflect both the increasing pro-portion of health discourse that this kind of data represents and the relative ease with which such data can be accessed (ethical issues notwithstanding) by those starting out in this field. The chapter reviews work that has explored what this kind of data can reveal about different facets of illness experiences, the role that online spaces can play for people with different conditions, how people construct and maintain identities and communities online, and how authenticity can be conveyed.

Organizing the book in this way brings to life the idea that concepts, approaches, and frameworks can be applied to multiple data types to answer many types of questions. Consider, for example, the notion of 'face' in the analysis of interactional data. The concept was originally defined by Goffman as:

> the positive social value a person effectively claims for himself [*sic*] by the line others assume he has taken during a particular contact. Face is an image of self delineated in terms of approved social attributes.
>
> *(Goffman, 1967: 5)*

This concept was developed in the prototypical context of face-to-face verbal interactions. However, Mullany et al. (2015) use the notion of face in a study of requests for advice about eating disorders sent by UK-based adolescents to the 'Virtual Surgery' of the health website 'Teenage Health Freaks' (Chapter 7) to explain why teenagers often attribute the belief that they are anorexic to their friends. They notice that requests for a diagnosis tend to include references to what other people say about the person's condition:

hello, in 13 and a male and like my friends all say i'm anorexic and all this rubbish and i'm not i must admit i feel so fat and ugly. i swim m many times a week but i just i don't no most of the people are so thin and mustly i'm 7 stone 3 pounds and i don't know if i am but i really do want to loose wait but i still eat stuff :(help!

(Mullany et al., 2015: 219)

Mullany et al. suggest that the sender of this message partly protects their own face in requesting advice by attributing the belief that they are anorexic to their friends ('my friends all say'), rather than taking direct responsibility for that claim.

Similarly, in a non-digital context, exploring representations of the experience of autism-spectrum disorders in fiction (Chapter 5), Semino (2014) looks at how Jessica, the protagonist of Clare Morrall's novel *The Language of Others*, interacts when meeting her boyfriend's parents (Miranda and Donald) for the first time in a restaurant. In one extract, after describing that they have 'admired' from a distance the dilapidated stately home in which Jessica's family live, Miranda adds that they 'went up the drive – just a little way – to have a peep. It's beautiful, isn't it?' (61–62). To this Jessica responds with 'It's a private drive'. The concept of face allows Semino to show why this response might be problematic and to highlight what aspect of communication – predicting and avoiding potential sources of friction in conversation – Jessica finds challenging.

Concepts and frameworks developed or prototypically used for one type of data, setting, or question, can successfully be applied to others – within reason, of course, as discussed in Chapter 2. The same is true for how you read the example studies in Part II of the book.

Part III concludes the volume with five case studies demonstrating challenges that can emerge during the life course of research projects (from identifying a research focus to data analysis) and how these can be addressed. Each chapter draws on one or more of the authors' own experiences and intimate knowledge of research projects on a variety of topics. Chapter 9 showcases a study on medical advertising to show how complex social phenomena can be studied on a small scale. Chapter 10 focuses on metaphors for Covid-19 and outlines how there can be many different sources of inspiration for research questions and what you can do when some of your questions cannot be answered with the data you have. In Chapter 11 we explore the role of pro-vaccination narratives in discussions of vaccine hesitancy online and demonstrate how you can find a specific focus within a large dataset. Chapter 12 highlights a study exploring authenticity in role play tasks used in medical education and assessment, and demonstrates how every analytic step can emerge from and build on previous ones, as well as how real impact can be achieved with linguistics projects. Finally, Chapter 13 showcases a study of inter-professional communication in Schwartz Rounds to demonstrate how complex ethical issues for collecting and analyzing sensitive data can be addressed during a relatively short research project. These chapters aim to demystify the research process and make clear that the reality of research will always diverge from the plans and ideals, but that this is not something to be afraid of. In this way, we aim to inspire and embolden all our readers to begin and continue researching language and health.

Further readings

Brookes, G., & Hunt, D. (2021). *Analysing health communication: Discourse approaches.* Palgrave Macmillan.

Demjén, Z. (2020). *Applying linguistics in illness and healthcare contexts.* Bloomsbury.

Hamilton, H., & Chou, W. S. (2014). *The Routledge handbook of language and health communication.* Routledge.

Harvey, K., & Koteyko, N. (2013). *Exploring health communication: Language in action.* Routledge.

Penn, C., & Watermeyer, J. (2018). *Communicating across cultures and languages in the health care setting: Voices of care.* Palgrave Macmillan.

References

Boyd, E., & Heritage, J. (2006). Taking the history: Questioning during comprehensive history taking. In J. Heritage & D. W. Maynard (Eds.), *Communication in medical care: Interaction between primary care physicians and patients* (pp. 151–184). Cambridge University Press.

Brookes, G., Harvey, K., & Mullany, L. (2016). 'Off to the best start'? A multimodal critique of breast and formula feeding health promotional discourse. *Gender and Language, 10*(3), 340–363.

Bucholtz, M., & Hall, K. (2005). Identity and interaction: A sociocultural linguistic approach. *Discourse Studies, 7*(4–5), 585–614.

Collins, L. C., Jaspal, R., & Nerlich, B. (2018). Who or what has agency in the discussion of antimicrobial resistance in UK news media (2010–2015)? A transitivity analysis. *Health, 22*(6), 521–540.

Cummings, L. (2008). *Clinical linguistics.* Edinburgh University Press.

Goffman, E. (1967). *Interaction ritual: Essays on face-to-face interaction.* Aldine Publishing.

Harvey, K. (2012). Disclosures of depression: Using corpus linguistics methods to examine young people's online health concerns. *International Journal of Corpus Linguistics, 17*(3), 349–379.

Heritage, J., Robinson, J. D., Elliott, M. N., Beckett, M., & Wilkes, M. (2007). Reducing patients' unmet concerns in primary care: The difference one word can make. *Journal of General Internal Medicine, 22*(10), 1429–1433.

McInerney, S. J. (2002). Rapid response: Introducing the biopsychosocial model for good medicine and good doctors. *BMJ, 324*, 1537.

Mullany, L., Smith, C., Harvey, K., & Adolphs, S. (2015). 'Am I anorexic?' weight, eating and discourses of the body in online adolescent health communication. *Communication and Medicine, 12*(2–3), 211–223.

Semino, E. (2014). Pragmatic failure, mind style and characterization in fiction about autism. *Language and Literature, 23*(2), 141–158.

Yuill, C., Crinson, I., & Duncan, E. (2010). The biomedical model of health. In Yuill, C., Crinson, I., & Duncan, E. (Eds.), *Key concepts in health studies* (pp. 7–10). Sage.

2
GETTING STARTED WITH RESEARCH
Questions, data, methods

2.1 Introduction

Doing a project on language and communication in healthcare can be one of the most rewarding experiences in your studies or research career. Our students often tell us that they did not expect to have the option to research a health-related topic from a linguistic perspective, and that they enjoyed the process and were eventually proud of what they achieved. However, as in any other area of research, it is not straightforward to go from an interest in or concern for a particular condition or healthcare setting to outlining a viable project and carrying it out successfully. For example, you may have an interest in communication about eating disorders, but how do you turn that interest into a worthwhile, viable, and successful research project?

This chapter takes you through the decisions and processes that you will have to engage in while going from that initial interest to a completed project that you can write about in a piece of coursework, dissertation, or thesis, namely: choosing a topic area; formulating research questions; identifying and collecting data; and selecting and applying research methods. At each stage, we will consider the options you may have, the decisions you will have to make, the pitfalls you should try to avoid, and the work you will have to do.

While we are concerned with empirical, data-focused studies of communication about illness, the issues we discuss apply in similar ways to doing research in Linguistics and Discourse Analysis more generally, as well as beyond. Alongside the advice and support available in your college or university, you may therefore find it useful to consult general textbooks on research methods in (applied) Linguistics, such as Wray and Bloomer (2012) and Litoselliti (2018).

DOI: 10.4324/9781003020417-3

2.2 Choosing a topic area

We begin by discussing the process of selecting a topic area for a research project on some aspect of language and health. To come to a decision, you will need to consider and balance several different perspectives: personal, academic, contextual, and practical.

2.2.1 Personal considerations

It is crucial that you find the topic of your research project interesting and meaningful, because you will have to devote a lot of time and effort to it. In fact, at some point in the course of the research and writing, you may well get to hate your topic (hopefully, not for a long time), which makes it even more important that you are passionate about it to begin with.

In practice, this may mean that you will consider working on a health-related topic that you have some personal experience of. There is, however, an important balance to be struck in your personal involvement with the topic. Let us take eating disorders as an example. If you have never experienced eating disorders, whether directly or as a friend or relative, nor had the chance to read or hear about them before, you would be starting from a considerable distance from your topic, and may well decide to study something else. Conversely, if you or someone close to you is currently very seriously affected by an eating disorder, you may be too close to the topic. That could increase the risk that you will find data collection and analysis distressing – a phenomenon known as 'vicarious trauma' – and/or that you will struggle to approach your data as a researcher, rather than someone who is deeply involved with the experiences reflected in your data (see also Chapter 3, section 3.6). In other words, the distance between you and the topic should ideally be neither too large nor too small. You may, for example, be close to someone who has had difficulties due to an eating disorder in the past, but you may start your project when that person is reasonably well and happy. That way, the distance between you and the topic may be 'just right'. Nonetheless, you will always want to be mindful of how you may be affected by analyzing, for example, first-person narratives by people with eating disorders. This applies generally to any project about experiences and data that may cause upset or distress.

2.2.2 Academic considerations

Any research project should aim to fill a 'gap' in what is already known about a particular topic. That is what makes a project original and worth pursuing from a research point of view. The gap is likely to be a small one, but it needs to be clearly identifiable, and the way in which it can be identified is by carrying out a literature review to determine what is already known about the topic.[1] For example, you may discover that several studies have investigated the use of metaphors to describe the experience of eating disorders in different types of data (e.g.

Bates, 2015, Senkbeil & Hoppe, 2016), but that no study has yet looked at metaphors and anorexia on a particular social media platform that you are familiar with, or multimodal metaphors in a graphic novel about bulimia that you have found interesting. That could constitute the gap that your project aims to fill.

2.2.3 Contextual considerations

The choice of a research topic may also be driven by topicality or urgency at a particular point. For example, a celebrity's revelation that they are experiencing an eating disorder may cause reactions in the mainstream media and social media that you could decide to investigate. Or, more broadly, new statistics revealing an increase in anxiety disorders among students in Higher Education might lead you to carry out a study of first-person accounts of anxiety in your own university. In Chapter 10 we talk about a study on metaphors for Covid-19 that one of the authors of this book carried out in the first phase of the pandemic, in response to public debates at the time on the use of metaphors by politicians, scientists, and journalists.

2.2.4 Practical considerations

Last but not least, any research project has to be realistic and feasible, given your circumstances, previous experience and the time you have available. For example, recording and analyzing interactions between healthcare professionals and people with eating disorders in a specialist clinic would be a very interesting project, but it may in practice not be feasible in the space of a few months, because of difficulties of access and the length of the process of ethical approval (see Chapter 3). Similarly, it may be unrealistic to plan a project involving the use of Corpus Linguistics methods if you have never been trained in those methods before. We will return to these considerations in the course of the chapter.

Overall, therefore, the topic area you choose for your project should be:

- Meaningful to you, but not so personally close to make the research difficult;
- Original enough to fill a gap in the literature;
- Relevant at the time of the research, or even particularly timely and urgent;
- Feasible based on the time you have and your own expertise.

2.3 Formulating research questions

Once you have identified your general topic area, you are in a position to formulate one or more research questions that your study will aim to answer. That can feel like a daunting task, however, especially if you don't have much experience of developing research questions.

A literature review, and discussions with your tutors or supervisors, will help you establish the 'gap' in knowledge that your research questions aim to fill. In addition, an appropriate research question has been defined as 'one that you can envisage finding an answer to' (Wray & Bloomer, 2012: 1). More precisely, it needs to be formulated in such a way that there is 'a way of addressing it, in terms of identifying the appropriate data, collecting it and analysing it' (Sunderland, 2018: 20).

Let us consider some concrete examples of possible questions one may formulate in the area of eating disorders.

1. *How effective is cognitive-behavioural therapy for young people with anorexia?*
   This is a very important question, but it is not a linguistic question. If you are reading this book, you are likely to be interested in language and Linguistics, so you need to consider whether you have the theoretical grounding and methodological expertise required to answer this question.
2. *How are metaphors used in cognitive-behavioural therapy sessions about anorexia?*
   This is a viable and worthwhile linguistic question but, before planning a study around it, you need to check that you are able to get access to a sufficient number of recordings of therapy sessions, or transcripts of those sessions, in a specific setting within the timescales of your project. Ethics approval is likely to be more complex for interactions in healthcare settings and may take longer to obtain than for other types of data (see Chapter 3).
3. *Do people with anorexia use metaphors on 'X' social media platforms to describe their experiences?*
   This question relates to an interesting topic but is inappropriately formulated as a yes/no interrogative. As metaphor is a frequent phenomenon, particularly in the representation of illness, the answer is very unlikely to be 'no'. However, answering this question with a 'yes' does not, strictly speaking, tell us anything particularly interesting from the linguistic perspective taken in this book. This is in contrast with the kind of experimental research (not covered in this book) that focuses on the testing of hypotheses (e.g. on the outcomes of particular interventions), where yes/no questions are appropriate.
4. *How do people with anorexia use metaphors on 'X' social media platforms to describe their experiences?*
   This kind of question is usually a viable starting point for a project in Linguistics and Discourse Analysis, assuming you already have some experience of metaphor analysis: it can be answered using linguistic analysis; it involves data that is in the public domain (although you would still need to consider the ethical issues described in Chapter 3); and it focuses on the 'how' of language use, which enables you both to describe patterns in your data and to interpret them.

Let us imagine that you have decided on research question 4 for your project, that you have considered relevant ethical issues, and secured ethical approval for data collection and analysis. You will still find that the question is rather too general for the purposes of your analysis. To focus your study, you will still need to identify a relevant and manageable dataset from your chosen social media platform, and formulate more specific research questions.

For example, you may identify a thread on the social media platform where the first post encourages people to respond to the prompt 'For me, anorexia is … ' and discover that, at that particular point in time, there are 150 replies to that first post, many of which include metaphorical description of anorexia. You could decide to focus your analysis on that thread, and develop more specific questions to help you answer question 4 above, such as:

a) What kinds of metaphors are used to describe the experience of anorexia?
b) What aspects of anorexia are captured by the different kinds of metaphor? (e.g. self-perceptions, relationship with food, relationships with other people.)
c) What are the most frequent patterns in metaphor use? (i.e. based on both (a) and (b) above.)
d) What framings are suggested by the most frequent patterns of metaphor use? (e.g. in terms of the agency and empowerment or disempowerment of the person with anorexia; Semino et al., 2018.)
e) What are the implications of the findings for support and counselling?

At this point, question (4) above could be described as your 'overarching' research question, and (a) to (e) as a selection of specific research questions you could apply to your chosen dataset in order to be able to answer the overarching question. The number of specific research questions you have will depend on the scope of your study (e.g. Undergraduate dissertation or PhD thesis).

In practice, research questions tend to be refined and adjusted as the research progresses, but they have an important function, especially when operating under tight timeframes: they guide the collection and analysis of the data, and they keep you focused. The more you become familiar with your data, the more you will notice other interesting things you could investigate (e.g. the use of negation or storytelling). These may all be worthwhile in principle, but, if they are not relevant to your research questions, they need to be set aside for future research directions, which you can mention in the conclusions to your study. Remaining focused on your research questions is necessary to complete your project on time.

2.4 Identifying and collecting data

The data you will collect and analyze for a project on language and health, or for any other project, needs to be:

• Relevant to your research question(s);
• Feasible to collect in terms of practical access and by obtaining relevant ethical approval in good time;

- Possible to analyze in the time you have and using methods you are familiar with, or can become familiar with, so that you can answer your research question(s).

In this section we consider the main types of data that are relevant to studies on language and health, in increasing order of complexity of associated issues of access and ethics. As we do so, we will refer forward to sections in the book where we discuss studies that have used each type of data.

2.4.1 Published literature and other media

The experience of illness can be the focus of published works such as novels, comic strips, autobiographies and collections of poems, as well as films, TV or radio series, and podcasts. Whether fictional or otherwise, such works can provide powerful representations of the lived experience of different types of conditions, which can in turn play a major role in general perceptions and public debates. In Chapter 5 we discuss studies of, for example, the fictional representation of dementia (Harrison, 2017) and an autobiographical account of voice-hearing in the context of psychosis (Demjén & Semino, 2015). Although you may, in some cases, have to consider copyright issues (explained in Chapter 3), published works are, by definition, in the public domain. They are therefore accessible and do not require that you obtain consent from the authors to carry out your study. Some colleges/universities may nonetheless require you to complete an ethics application.

2.4.2 Press reports

In spite of the rise of social media, newspapers are still a major part of public discourse and a major reflection of and influence on public opinion, whether they are read in print or online. You may therefore be interested in studying how different kinds or aspects of illness and healthcare are represented in the press. In Chapter 4, for example, we discuss a study (Collins et al., 2018) of how the UK press represents antimicrobial resistance (i.e. resistance to antibiotics) – one of the ten major threats to global health identified by the World Health Organization in 2019. Datasets of news articles can be created fairly straightforwardly, including from digital databases and collections that may be available from your institution's library. This kind of data also does not require that you obtain consent from the authors to carry out your study. Some institutions may nonetheless require you to complete an ethics application.

2.4.3 Public health campaign materials

Public health messages can be disseminated through many different kinds of media, including the press (above) and social media (below). You may also be interested, however, in studying 'self-standing' public health materials such as billboards, posters, leaflets, or public service announcements on TV. In Chapter 4, for example, we discuss a study focusing on a poster campaign for HIV prevention in Nigeria (Oyebode & Unuabonah, 2013). Such materials are in the public domain and usually fairly straightforward to access and reproduce to a sufficiently high standard for inclusion in an essay or dissertation. You will still need to consider the specifics of the contexts and the organizations and agencies involved, however, in order to determine matters of consent and the nature of ethical approval you might require (see Chapter 3).

2.4.4 Online communication and social media

Online sources and interactions play an increasingly important part in the experience of illness and the practice of healthcare, and therefore offer a wide range of opportunities for research on language and health. In Chapter 7, for example, we discuss several studies of how advice about a range of health conditions is sought and provided on different online services for young people (e.g. Locher, 2006, Mullany et al., 2015). In Chapter 8, we describe research on how people with cancer forge community bonds through the use of humorous metaphors on an online forum (Semino et al., 2018).

Data from online sources varies in terms of how easy it is to collect, and you will need to consider what is feasible for you in the time you have. For example, a study on a selection of blog posts on the experience of Obsessive Compulsive Disorder does not require any specialized expertise in terms of data collection. In contrast, collecting tweets through the API that, at the time of writing, Twitter provides for researchers (https://developer.twitter.com/en/products/twitter-api/academic-research) involves several stages and some technical know-how. You need to explore what is feasible based on your own skills and the support you have available before embarking on a study that may involve, for example, the creation of a large corpus of tweets.

With regard to ethics, a project on, for example, the website of a governmental health agency involves no issues of permission, but any data drawn from what people write online as private individuals does raise questions about the appropriate level of consent and ethics approval. If you are considering collecting data from blogs, vlogs, online forums, or social media platforms, in Chapter 3 we provide a guide to the issues you will need to consider, depending on the precise data sources you have in mind (e.g. a named individual's blog vs. a publicly accessible online forum) and the analysis you plan to carry out (e.g. a qualitative analysis involving lengthy verbatim quotations vs. a corpus linguistic analysis mainly involving the presentation of quantitative findings).

2.4.5 Interactions in healthcare settings

Much of our experience of healthcare involves conversations with healthcare professionals, whether in a shared physical setting or, as is increasingly the case, through a digital platform. The successful provision of healthcare also involves interactions among healthcare professionals themselves. Studying such interactions from a linguistic perspective has a long tradition and contributes to answering very important research questions. Chapter 6 is entirely dedicated to this type of data. For example, we discuss research on how best to elicit from patients information about additional health concerns before the end of a consultation (Heritage et al., 2007), and on how relationships of power and authority can be negotiated, and sometimes subverted, in interactions between parents and doctors in paediatric consultations (Stivers, 2002).

In Chapters 3 and 6, we emphasize how issues of access and ethics often make it unrealistic to aim to collect new data from healthcare setting interactions in the time that is usually available for Undergraduate or Master-level projects, although it can be feasible in the context of doctoral research. Before committing to any such plans for data collection, you therefore need to give some serious consideration to these issues, and discuss them with your advisors. It may, however, be possible to have access to recordings or transcripts as part of larger projects at the institution where you are studying. In Chapter 6 we also provide some indication of where or how it is possible to access publicly available recordings of healthcare interactions that may be suitable for the research questions you aim to answer.

2.5 Selecting and applying research methods

Decisions about what methods to apply in your research depend on your own expertise and on the interaction between your data and your research questions.

With regard to your expertise, a research project provides an opportunity to play to your strengths and apply some of the methods that you have become familiar with in the course of your studies, and that, ideally, you have evidence that you are good at. This may involve going deeper into areas you have already studied and practised, as opposed to learning something completely new from scratch. For example, you may already have some expertise in using the methods associated with Corpus Linguistics – the computer-aided linguistic analysis of large datasets (see below), and you may learn how to use new or more sophisticated corpus techniques in order to carry out your project. If, however, you are not familiar with corpus methods at all, it is likely to be unrealistic or even risky to attempt to learn them and apply them over the usually short timeframes of a coursework project or an Undergraduate or Master's dissertation.

Once you have taken into account your own expertise and aptitude, you will need to consider what methods are most appropriate to answer your research questions by analyzing the data you have available or aim to collect. This is the golden triangle we mentioned in Chapter 1 (reproduced in Figure 2.1).

The rest of this section is structured according to broad distinctions between data types: interactional data, non-interactional data, multimodal data, and large quantities of data. In each sub-section, we briefly introduce the methods that are most appropriate to each data type, depending on the specific research questions.

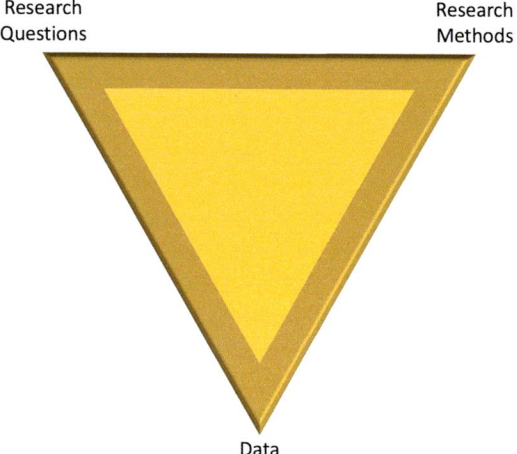

Research
Questions

Research
Methods

Data

FIGURE 2.1   The golden triangle of Research Questions, Methods, and Data

Each of those methods will receive more attention and exemplification in the course of the book. The final sub-section includes some considerations that apply across different methods and data types.

2.5.1 Interactional data

Many different types of interactional data are potentially relevant to studies on language and health, including:

- Spoken interactions in healthcare settings, whether in person or mediated through technology, e.g. GP or specialist consultations, therapy sessions, and handover conversations between nurses (see Chapter 6);
- Synchronous or asynchronous online interactions about illness, e.g. via email or messaging platforms, online advice sites, and peer-to-peer online forums dedicated to different health topics (see Chapters 7 and 8);
- Literary or fictional representations of the above, e.g. plays or stretches of dialogue in novels where the protagonist has dementia or an autism-spectrum disorder (see Chapter 5).

If your data is originally spoken, you need to adopt a transcription method that is appropriate for your study, i.e. such that you can analyze your data for the phenomena you are interested in and reproduce extracts in the write-up of your project. As we show in more detail in Chapter 6, different kinds of transcription are appropriate for different projects.

To analyze your data, you will then have to apply methods drawn from one or more of the broad areas of Linguistics and cognate areas that are concerned with how people interact with one another, whether those interactions are fictional or real, and whether they occur in speech or in writing. These areas include: Conversation Analysis, Interactional Sociolinguistics, Pragmatics, as well as Linguistic and Digital Ethnography.

Conversation Analysis aims to reveal patterns in people's oral interactions by describing in detail and in a 'bottom-up' fashion observable features of ongoing talk (ten Have, 2007). This involves a particularly detailed approach to the transcription of speech (described in Chapter 6) that captures phenomena such as pauses, overlaps, and loudness, in addition to the words spoken. Conversation Analysis has been applied, for example, to study the answers that tend to be elicited by particular types of questions in health professional-patient interactions. A study outlined in Chapter 6 demonstrates that when patients are asked if they have 'any other' concerns towards the end of a consultation, they are more likely to answer negatively than if they are asked if they have 'some other' concerns. This is because the use of 'any' suggests the expectation of a 'no' answer, whereas 'some' does not, with implications for how we train healthcare professionals (Heritage et al., 2007). Conversation Analysis has been applied particularly in analyzing the sequences of actions that unfold during the phases of medical consultations, from openings, history taking, diagnoses through to treatment decisions. A later example in Chapter 6, for example, illustrates the application of Conversation Analysis to reveal how patients and caregivers can negotiate their preferred prescription outcomes, challenging the asymmetry and power-imbalance we typically imagine of the doctor–patient relationship.

Interactional sociolinguistics is similarly concerned with the detailed description of spoken interactions, but has a greater focus on the wider social and cultural context in which those interactions take place, particularly where there may be differences in the linguistic resources available to speakers (Gumperz, 1999). It has been extensively employed in institutional settings, like healthcare, where the power and identity of speakers become negotiated in the interaction. For example, in Chapter 6 we discuss a series of studies by Zayts and Schnurr (2014) on genetic counselling interactions between nurses and patients or family members in Hong Kong. Zayts and Schnurr show how the nurses alternate between different roles in relation to their interlocutors (e.g. medical professional, counsellor, cultural broker) and explain this alternation with reference to the multicultural and multilingual setting of Hong Kong, and the diversity of the people who seek genetic counselling.

Pragmatics is a broad area that is concerned with how meanings are constructed and relationships negotiated through the ways in which people interact in context (Culpeper & Haugh, 2014). Key concepts within Pragmatics include:

- 'speech acts' – the actions we perform via speaking or writing (Austin, 1962);
- Grice's (1975) 'Cooperative Principle' and 'Conversational Maxims' – the implicit assumptions that explain how we often mean more than we say or infer more than is said;
- 'face' – our public image (Goffmann, 1967);
- '(im)politeness' or 'rapport-management' – the ways in which we manage our own and others' faces in attempting to achieve our interactional goals (Brown and Levinson, 1987, Spencer-Oatey, 2008, Culpeper, 2011).

Methods drawn from Pragmatics can be used, for example, to answer questions about how people manage advice-seeking and advice-giving in health-related interactions. In Chapter 7 we discuss a study by Locher (2010) that shows how 'mitigation' strategies such as hedges are used on an online health advice column for students to reduce the potential face threat (or danger of causing offence) associated with advice-giving. In Chapter 5 we show how concepts from Pragmatics can be used to answer questions about the construction of characters in fiction. This applies, for example, to cases where the fact that a character repeatedly but unintentionally causes face damage to other characters may be interpreted as evidence of an autism-spectrum disorder (Semino, 2014).

Ethnography similarly captures a broad area that lies at the interface between Linguistics and Anthropology, with the field of 'Linguistic Ethnography' coming to prominence in the past couple of decades (Copland & Creese, 2015). What is distinctive about ethnographic approaches is that the researcher observes or even becomes involved in the group and activities they aim to study, drawing the perspectives of participants and their understandings of the social groups they inhabit. Analysis is therefore interpretive and involves not only closely studying the *products* of communication (e.g. texts and images), but also incorporates an understanding of the social *processes* and *practices* from which those products arise and which they work to shape. Ethnographies can involve studying the practices of particular ethnic, social, or cultural groups but also particular settings, such as institutional ethnographies of workplace communication, like healthcare. In healthcare settings such as GP clinics, this can be very challenging, due to issues of access, safety, and confidentiality, although some students do find opportunities to do this type of research (see Chapter 3 for further details on fieldwork ethics). In Chapter 8 we provide an example of 'digital' ethnography, where researchers addressed a series of questions about the constructions of identities by observing, over a period of four months, the Facebook accounts of 20 people with type 1 and type 2 diabetes (Koteyko & Hunt, 2016).

2.5.2 Non-interactional data

Depending on your research questions, a range of different approaches may be relevant to the analysis of non-interactional data, which includes health information websites, news reports, novels, autobiographies, and so on. Here we consider concepts and frameworks associated with Critical Discourse Analysis and Stylistics.

Critical Discourse Analysis (CDA; Wodak & Meyer, 2009) is particularly relevant to questions concerning the role of ideologies in the representation of people associated with different health conditions, and the perpetuation of stigma and power inequalities. Different approaches within CDA apply different analytical frameworks to study, for example, how individuals and groups are labelled, how entities and behaviours are evaluated, and how agency, responsibility, and blame are attributed. A study we discuss in Chapter 4 (Mulderrig, 2017) considers the linguistic strategies used in an anti-obesity TV advertisement in contrast with official reports and policy documents from the UK government. The study shows how the ad emphasizes personal responsibility for obesity, as opposed to social determinants, via linguistic strategies such as exaggeration, emotive lexis, and vagueness in the use of the first-person plural pronoun 'we'.

Stylistics lies at the interface between Linguistics and Literary Studies and is concerned with how linguistic choices are used to achieve a range of effects that are particularly relevant to the study of fiction and literature, such as the construction of characters and the representation of different points of view (Jeffries & McIntyre, 2010). Stylistic approaches can be relevant to this book when they are used to answer questions about the representation of the experience of illness and of characters with particular conditions, as well as the potential influence of such representations on public perceptions and debates. In Chapter 5 we discuss a study by Demjén and Semino (2015) that focuses on the presentation of speech in an autobiographical account of the hearing of voices that others cannot hear (or auditory verbal hallucinations) by a young man called Henry Cockburn. In Stylistics, different ways of presenting the speech of characters in fictional narratives (e.g. through Direct Speech or Indirect Speech) are known to play a part in the construction of those characters (Leech & Short, 2007). Demjén and Semino point out differences in how Henry's presents 'hallucinatory' vs. 'real' voices, and suggest that this may reflect subtle differences in how he experiences these different kinds of voices.

Both CDA and Stylistics also draw from different areas of Linguistics to achieve their goals. These include, for example, Systemic Functional Linguistics (Halliday, 1994), Cognitive Linguistics (Langacker, 2008), Conceptual Metaphor Theory (Lakoff & Johnson, 1980) and some of the areas we have already mentioned, such as Pragmatics. With regard to Stylistics, in Chapter 5 we discuss a study of the fictional representation of the experience of dementia that uses concepts from Cognitive Linguistics (Harrison, 2017), and an analysis of the fictional representation of autism that draws from Pragmatics to explain how the perception of a character as autistic may result from the ways in which they are presented as interacting with other characters in the course of a novel (Semino, 2014).

The variety of specific analytical frameworks associated with different areas of Linguistics and Discourse Analysis provides further opportunities for you to build on your strengths and interests in selecting the precise methods to be adopted in your study.

2.5.3 Multimodal data

If your project focuses on a novel, as in the study by Harrison (2017), you are dealing with just one mode of making meaning, i.e. writing. However, many other types of data are 'multi-modal', i.e. involve more than one mode. For example, a face-to-face medical consultation minimally involves speech and gesture; a poster about a flu vaccination campaign may involve writing and visual choices in terms of font, layout, and images; and in news articles and tweets, images, and video clips or GIFs often accompany the written text.

Depending on your access to data and your research questions, you may have good reasons for analyzing a single mode of communication in data that is in fact multimodal. For example, your access to a face-to-face medical consultation may be limited to an audio-recording, or your research questions may be answerable by analyzing transcripts such as those discussed in the previous section, which capture only speech, at different levels of detail. Similarly, your research questions may be concerned with how particular groups of people (e.g. people with heart failure or dementia) are represented in a press corpus that contains a large number of articles (e.g. tens of thousands of texts, amounting to millions of words) but omits any images that may have accompanied those articles in the printed or online versions of the relevant newspapers.

On the other hand, it may be possible and necessary to consider the different modes involved in your data, both individually and in interaction with each other. The areas of Multimodality and Social Semiotics, which are central to some strands of Critical Discourse Analysis, focus on how meanings arise from the interaction of different modes in particular communicative contexts. Kress and Van Leeuwen's (2006) visual grammar is a highly influential approach to the analysis of images and multimodal texts, as we show in Chapters 4 and 9. This approach accounts for the different ways in which entities, relationships, and processes can be represented visually, and makes it possible to discuss the implications of different choices. A study we discuss in Chapter 4, for example (Brookes et al., 2016), points out a contrast in photographs of breastfeeding vs. bottle-feeding mothers in guides produced by the UK's National Health Service, for example in terms of gaze. Breastfeeding mothers are portrayed at eye level with the viewer, while bottle-feeding mothers are portrayed as looking away from the viewer. This makes it easier to experience closeness and intimacy with mothers who breastfeed, in contrast with those who bottle feed.

While not covered in this book, some studies of interactions in healthcare settings combine detailed phonetic or prosodic analyses with frameworks derived from Conversation Analysis or Pragmatics. For example, Vickers and Goble (2018) studied interactions between nurses and patients in a bilingual (English-Spanish) community clinic in California. They showed how different communicative styles on the part of the health professionals ('authoritarian' vs. 'egalitarian') are constructed via different patterns of choice in terms of politeness (from the domain of Pragmatics) and prosodic cues, such as pitch and intonation (analyzed via the software Praat). Vickers and Gable also consider the implications of different communicative styles for relationships between nurses and patients, and for subsequent patient health outcomes.

2.5.4 Large quantities of verbal data

Depending on your research questions and the size of the data you intend to analyze, you may need to draw from the methods of Corpus Linguistics. This involves using tailor-made software to study digitally stored collections of texts known as 'corpora'.

Corpus methods are relevant when the data needed to answer your research questions is, as McEnery and Hardie (2012: 1–2) put it, 'of a size which defies analysis by hand and eye alone within any reasonable timeframe'. Although there is no definite cut-off point in this respect, corpus-based studies of topics relevant to this book tend to involve datasets consisting of millions of words. For example, Mullany et al. (2015) analyzed a 2-million-word corpus of teenagers' requests for advice on weight and eating, while Brookes and Baker (2017) use a range of corpus methods to study a 29-million-word corpus of feedback on NHS services (Brookes & Baker, 2017). The study of press representations of particular health-related issues also typically involve the use of corpus methods, as Collins et al.'s (2018) analysis of a corpus consisting of 627 articles from 16 UK national newspapers that included the words 'antibiotic resistance', 'antimicrobial resistance', or 'superbug' between 2010 and 2015 (see Chapter 4).

Several suites of corpus tools are available for free, such as AntConc (www.laurenceanthony.net/software/antconc/), CQPWeb (https://cqpweb.lancs.ac.uk), and #LancsBox (http://corpora.lancs.ac.uk/lancsbox/). Others require an individual or institutional subscription, but may be available to you via your college or university, such as Sketchengine (www.sketchengine.eu), WordsSmith Tools (www.lexically.net/wordsmith/), and Wmatrix (https://ucrel-wmatrix4.lancaster.ac.uk). While there are differences in how you access and use each of these pieces of software, they all make it possible to carry out the most well established types of analysis in Corpus Linguistics, which involve frequencies, keyness comparisons, concordances, and collocations (see also Baker, 2018).

Frequencies – As we discuss in Chapter 7, Baker et al. (2019) analyzed a 29-million word corpus of online feedback on NHS services writing, in order to answer questions about what was evaluated positively or negatively by patients and why. One of their ways into the data was to extract from the corpus a 'frequency list', i.e. a list of all words in the corpus in descending order of frequency. Baker et al. then identified the ten most frequent words that expressed positive evaluation (e.g. 'excellent') and the ten most frequent words that expressed negative evaluation (e.g. 'terrible'). This enabled them to compare the overall frequencies of the positive vs. negative evaluative words, and to discover that, cumulatively, the positive words were about three times more frequent than the negative words. For the purposes of their study, it was appropriate to work with 'absolute' frequencies, i.e. the total number of occurrences of evaluative words. If your goal is to compare corpora of different sizes, however, you will need to consider relative frequencies (e.g. occurrences per 1,000 words), which are also provided by corpus software.

Keyness comparisons – A different corpus technique that can provide a useful way into your data is keyness analysis. This involves using corpus tools that compare the relative frequencies of words in one dataset (the 'target' corpus) with those in another dataset (the 'reference' corpus). The output of the tool is a list of words ('keywords') that are used much more frequently, relative to the size of each corpus, in the target corpus than in the reference corpus. In Corpus Linguistics, therefore, keywords are words that are characteristic of a specific corpus of interest as compared with an appropriate reference corpus, and that therefore capture the 'aboutness' of a particular corpus (Scott, 1997). As we discuss in Chapter 7, for example, Mullany et al. compared a corpus of requests for online health advice by teenagers with a general corpus of English, in order to begin to identify the main health concerns that prompted the requests for advice (e.g. keywords relating to eating and eating disorders, such as 'dieting', 'vegan', and 'anorexia'). Different corpus tools provide different options for the statistical measures to be adopted to decide what counts as a keyword. In Chapters 7 and 8 we also discuss studies using corpus tools that make it possible to carry out keyness analyses not just at the word level, but also at the level of parts of speech (e.g. all pronouns considered together) and of semantic fields (e.g. all words relating to medicine together).

Concordance analyses – When you have identified a set of words or phrases that you are interested in, whether because of their frequencies, keyness status or other reasons, you may use a 'concordancing' tool to search for all instances of those words/phrases and see each of them on a separate line, with the words that precede and follow each instance (as in Figure 2.2, where KWIC stands for 'Key Word in Context'). This makes it possible to study qualitatively how those words/phrases are used in context. For example, in Chapter 7 we discuss how Harvey (2012) analyzed concordances for the phrases 'I am depressed' and 'I have depression' in requests for health advice and found a difference in the kind of problem that was written about depending on which phrase was used.

Collocations – A different approach to studying the context in which words or phrases occur is made possible by corpus tools that produce rank-ordered lists of words (known as 'collocates') that occur with distinctively high frequencies around the word/phrase of interest. For example, Baker et al. (2019) studied the collocates of the 20 most frequent words expressing positive or negative evaluation in their corpus of feedback on NHS services. This enabled them to identify the main aspects of health services that the feedback was about, and to note that healthcare staff's interpersonal skills was the aspect that was most frequently commented on, whether positively or negatively (e.g. collocates such as 'manner' and 'attitude').

	Details	Left context	KWIC	Right context
1	freeread.com.au	'</s><s>He left the room presently.</s><s>The	nurse	was upon the threshold.</s><s>"Quite," he ans\
2	lifeflighteagle...	:s>Learn more about what it takes to be a flight	nurse	or flight paramedic.</s><s>Our medical teams ;
3	dva.gov.au	d.</s><s>He shifts under the blanket.</s><s>A	nurse	dresses a soldier's foot.</s><s>In full uniform, h
4	philippinesusa....	nd we are acting on this: In 2010, ten thousand	nurses	and midwives were deployed under the RNHeal
5	vic.gov.au	mediate, expert health advice from a registered	nurse	, 24 hours a day, 7 days a week for the cost of a
6	docplayer.net	g Certified Nursing Assisting Licensed Practical	Nurse	Registered Nurse Medical Assistant Optometris
7	columbia.edu	to inform healthcare and health policy.</s><s>	Nurses	will play all types of roles in healthcare, some w
8	wondersandmarve...	ctive nurses.</s><s>She pronounced all of the	nurses	suitable except for Hancock, whom she objecte‹
9	pomc.com	sloving a murder case. i have evidence that the	nurse	murder my husband on july 11,2001. i found ne\
10	authorsden.com	ess.</s><s>She dedicated her book to hospice	nurses	, and after its publication, became active in the ‹
11	rcn.org.uk	eview regarding research productivity amongst	nurse	academics.</s><s>Howden Suggers</s><s>SF
12	3-rx.com	en she started coughing," said Zahira Hussein,	nursing	her 13-month-old daughter in the feeding centre
13	ufhealth.org	ortant component will be placing a public health	nurse	on site - in a randomized clinical trial.</s><s>Tf
14	hcpro.com	TABS), that includes an interaction between the	nurse	whose shift is ending and the nurse whose shift
15	hopkinsmedicine...	ation, resources and support from a specialized	nurse	transition guide, in the hospital and at home.</s
16	vineyardgazette...	ing room or by letting her special care workers,	nurses	and doctors know how much they were needed
17	wikipedia.org	pital, Marie and Hasse are greeted by Martin, a	nurse	who specializes in care for patient's relatives.</
18	wikipedia.org	001, The Guardian noted that Britain had 3,000	nurses	specializing in breast cancer, compared to a sin
19	wikipedia.org	promoted twice: on first instance to senior staff	nurse	and on second instance to clinical nurse manag
20	wikipedia.org	one of the geriatric units of the hospital, where	nurses	hit and tied up elderly mentally ill patients, and r

FIGURE 2.2 Concordance of 'nurse' in EnTenTen20 created using SketchEngine (Kilgarriff et al., 2014)

Finally, Corpus Linguistics studies can also include the principled selection of a small subset of the data for detailed analysis. For example, at one point in their analysis of a 29-million-word corpus of feedback on NHS services, Brookes and Baker (2017) select for close reading a subset of 100 comments for each of the major themes they had previously identified in the data:

> To ensure that 100 comments provided a sufficiently representative sample for this stage in our analysis, we adopted a saturation point procedure, well established in such quantitative linguistic research, of randomly selecting 30 comments, analyzing the emergent patterns, proceeding to examine another 30 randomly selected comments and continuing the process until saturation point was reached and new patterns had ceased to emerge. New patterns, or drivers, were no longer emergent by the time we analyzed the 100th comment (positive and negative) for each theme, and so this sample

size was deemed sufficiently large to account for the common drivers of positive and negative feedback, yet small enough to facilitate fine-grain qualitative examination.

(Brookes & Baker, 2017: 3)

In Chapters 7 and 11 we provide further examples of how to 'zoom in' from a very large dataset to a sample that is small enough for a manual analysis.

2.5.5 Cross-cutting phenomena and operationalization

The areas we have discussed in the previous sections and their associated methodologies are not as separate as our overview may suggest. For example, corpus methods are often combined with detailed manual analyses of particular sections of the data, and Stylistics draws from Pragmatics and Conversation Analysis to explain how we perceive characters based on their conversational behaviour.

Some broad phenomena that you may be interested in can also be approached using the methods associated with different areas. For example, as noted in Chapter 1, in the course of the book we discuss several studies that focus on identities, whether in relation to patients, healthcare professionals, or other groups. These studies share what is known as a 'post-structuralist' view of identity, namely the idea that identities are not well defined and fixed characteristics of people, but, rather, are flexible, dynamic, context-dependent, and constructed and negotiated through discourse (Buchholz & Hall, 2005). Beyond this, however, one can approach identities by drawing from Conversation Analysis and Pragmatics (Chapter 6) as well as CDA and Ethnography (Chapter 8). Similarly, you may study the forms and functions of narratives and metaphors in health communication in different types of data and using different methods. For example, in Chapter 5 we discuss a study involving the manual qualitative analysis of multimodal metaphors for the experiences of cancer and depression in graphic novels (El Refaie, 2019), while in Chapter 8 we discuss a corpus-based study of metaphors for the experience of cancer in a 1.5-million-word corpus of interviews with and online forum posts by patients, family carers, and healthcare professionals (Semino et al., 2018).

Regardless of the approach you adopt, however, you will have to think and report exactly how you 'operationalize' the concepts that are central to your study. This involves providing definition of, for example, metaphor or narrative, drawing from the literature you have read, and also clarifying how you decide what counts as, for example, a reference to identities or an instance of a reference to a particular *type* of identity in your data. In many cases you will need to outline and follow a clear and replicable method for identifying the phenomena you are interested in. For example, in Chapter 8 the study by Semino et al. (2018) draws on the Metaphor Identification Procedure detailed in Pragglejaz Group (2007), while Chou et al. (2011) use Labov and Waletzky's (1967) classic framework to identify different components of YouTube narratives. The same applies to being clear and rigorous about how you group linguistic choices in your data under different categories, e.g. classifying keywords under different themes, or instances of metaphor under different categories. In the course of the book, we spell out how the authors of the studies we review have approached these difficult but necessary research steps.

2.6 Concluding remarks

In this chapter, we have provided a guide on how to go from an initial interest in a particular topic to the formulation of a viable and worthwhile research project. We have outlined the different considerations to be borne in mind when deciding on a topic. We have spelt out what makes an appropriate set of research questions. We have considered the processes and challenges involved in collecting different kinds of data. And we have outlined the areas of Linguistics that provide the main methods needed to analyze different kinds of data relevant to health communication. Our key message is that you need to make sure that you have a good fit between your research questions, your data, and your methods. In the course of the book, we will show how this tight fit has been achieved in many different studies on language and health. Before we do that, however, we need to give further consideration to the ethical dimension of conducting this kind of research. That is the topic of the next chapter.

Note

1 In health research, as well as other disciplines, there are different approaches to carrying out literature reviews, e.g. systematic reviews, meta-analyses, and so on (Aveyard et al., 2021). These distinctions are only beginning to be adopted in Linguistics, but it is always useful to check what is expected of you for a particular piece of work.

Further readings

Wray, A., & Bloomer, A. (2012). *Projects in linguistics and language studies* (3rd ed.). Routledge.

References

Austin, J. (1962). *How to do things with words*. Clarendon.
Aveyard, H., Payne, S., & Preston, N. (2021). *A post-graduate's guide to doing a literature review in health and social care* (2nd ed.). McGraw-Hill Education.
Bates, C. (2015). I am a waste of breath, of space, of time. *Qualitative Health Research*, 25(2), 189–204.
Baker, P. (2018). Corpus methods in linguistics. In L. Litosselliti (Ed.), *Research methods in linguistics* (2nd ed., 13–34). Continuum.
Baker, P., Brookes, G., & Evans, C. (2019). *The language of patient feedback: A corpus linguistic study of online health communication*. Routledge.

Brookes, G., & Baker, P. (2017). What does patient feedback reveal about the NHS? A mixed methods study of comments posted to the NHS Choices online service. *BMJ Open*, 7(4), E013821.

Brookes, G., Harvey, K., & Mullany, L. (2016). 'Off to the best start'? A multimodal critique of breast and formula feeding health promotional discourse. *Gender and Language*, 10(3), 340–363.

Brown, P., & Levinson, S. C. (1987). *Politeness: Some universals in language use*. Cambridge University Press.

Buchholz, M., & Hall, K. (2005). Identity and interaction: A sociocultural linguistic approach. *Discourse Studies*, 7(4–5), 585–614.

Chou, W.-Y. S., Hunt, Y., Folkers, A., & Augustson, E. (2011). Cancer survivorship in the age of YouTube and social media: A narrative analysis. *Journal of Medical Internet Research*, 13(1), 108–116.

Collins, L. C., Jaspal, R., & Nerlich, B. (2018). Who or what has agency in the discussion of antimicrobial resistance in UK news media (2010–2015)? A transitivity analysis. *Health*, 22(6), 521–540.

Copland, F., & Creese, A. (2015). *Linguistic ethnography: Collecting, analysing and presenting data*. Sage.

Culpeper, J. (2011). *Impoliteness: Using language to cause offence*. Cambridge University Press.

Culpeper, J., & Haugh, M. (2014). *Pragmatics and the English language*. Bloomsbury.

Demjén, Z., & Semino, E. (2015). Henry's voices: The representation of auditory verbal hallucinations in an autobiographical narrative. *Medical Humanities*, 41(1), 57–62.

El Refaie, E. (2019). *Visual metaphor and embodiment in graphic illness narratives*. Oxford University Press.

Goffman, E. (1967). *Interaction ritual: Essays on face-to-face interaction*. Aldine Publishing.

Grice, H. P. (1975). Logic and conversation. In P. Cole & J. L. Morgan (Eds.), *Syntax and semantics* (vol. 3, pp. 41–58). Academic Press.

Gumperz, J. (1999). On interactional sociolinguistic method. In S. Sarangi & C. Roberts (Eds.), *Talk, work, and institutional order: Discourse in medical, mediation, and management settings* (pp. 453–471). Mouton de Gruyter.

Halliday, M. A. K. (1994). *An introduction to functional grammar* (2nd ed.). Edward Arnold.

Harrison, C. (2017). Finding Elizabeth: Construing memory in Elizabeth is missing by Emma Healey. *Journal of Literary Semantics*, 46(2), 131–151.

Heritage, J., Robinson, J., Elliott, M., Beckett, M., & Wilkes, M. (2007). Reducing patients' unmet concerns in primary care: The difference one word can make. *Journal of General Internal Medicine*, 22(10), 1429–1433.

Harvey, K. (2012). Disclosures of depression: Using corpus linguistics methods to examine young people's online health concerns. *International Journal of Corpus Linguistics*, 17(3), 349–379.

Jeffries, L., & McIntyre, D. (2010). *Stylistics*. Cambridge University Press.

Kilgarriff, A., Baisa, V., Bušta, J., Jakubíček, M., Kovář, V., Michelfeit, J., Rychlý, P., Suchomel, V. (2014). The sketch engine: Ten years on. *Lexicography*, 1(1), 7–36.

Koteyko, N., & Hunt, D. (2016). Performing health identities on social media: An online observation of Facebook profiles. *Discourse, Context and Media*, 12, 59–67.

Kress, G., & van Leeuwen, T. (2006). *Reading images: The grammar of visual design*. Routledge.

Labov, W., & Waletzky, J. (1967 [1997]). Narrative analysis. In J. Helm (Ed.), *Essays on the verbal and visual arts* (pp. 12–44). University of Washington Press. Journal of Narrative and Life History, 7, 3–38.

Lakoff, G., & Johnson, M. (1980). *Metaphors we live by*. Chicago University Press.

Langacker, R. (2008). *Cognitive grammar: A basic introduction*. Oxford University Press.

Leech, G. N., & Short, M. H. (2007). *Style in fiction*. Longman.

Litosselliti, L. (ed.) (2018). *Research methods in linguistics* (2nd ed.). Continuum.

Locher, M. (2006). *Advice online: Advice-giving in an American Internet health column*. John Benjamins.

Locher, M. A. (2010). Health Internet sites: A linguistic perspective on health advice columns. *Social Semiotics, 20*(1), 43–59.

McEnery, T., & Hardie, A. (2012). *Corpus*. Cambridge University Press.

Mulderrig, J. (2017). Reframing obesity: a critical discourse analysis of the UK's first social marketing campaign, *Critical Policy Studies, 11*(4), 455–476.

Mullany, L., Smith, C., Harvey, K., & Adolphs, S. (2015). 'Am I anorexic?' weight, eating and discourses of the body in online adolescent health communication. *Communication and Medicine, 12*(2–3), 211–223.

Oyebode, O., & Unuabonah, F. O. (2013). Coping with HIV/AIDS: A multimodal discourse analysis of selected HIV/AIDS posters in south-western Nigeria. *Discourse and Society, 24*(6), 810–827.

Pragglejaz Group. (2007). MIP: A method for identifying metaphorically used words in discourse. *Metaphor and Symbol, 22*(1), 1–39.

Scott, M. (1997). PC analysis of key words - And key key words. *System, 25*(2), 233–245.

Semino, E. (2014). Pragmatic failure, mind style and characterization in fiction about autism. *Language and Literature, 23*(2), 141–158.

Semino, E., Demjén, Z., & Demmen, J. (2018). An integrated approach to metaphor and framing in cognition, discourse and practice, with an application to metaphors for cancer. *Applied Linguistics, 39*(5), 625–645.

Semino, E., Demjén, Z., Hardie, A., Rayson, P., & Payne, S. (2018). *Metaphor, cancer and the end of life: A corpus-based study*. Routledge.

Senkbeil, K., & Hoppe, N. (2016). 'The sickness stands at your shoulder …': Embodiment and cognitive metaphor in Hornbacher's wasted: A memoir of anorexia and bulimia. *Language and Literature, 25*(1), 3–17.

Spencer-Oatey, H. (2008). Rapport management: A framework for analysis. In H. Spencer-Oatey (Ed.), *Culturally speaking: Culture, communication and politeness theory* (2nd ed., pp. 11–47). Continuum.

Stivers, T. (2002). Participating in decisions about treatment: Overt parent pressure for antibiotic medication in pediatric encounters. *Social Science and Medicine, 54*(7), 1111–1130.

Sunderland, J. (2018). Research questions in linguistics. In L. Litosselliti (Ed.), *Research methods in linguistics* (2nd ed., 167–192). Continuum.

ten Have, P. (2007). *Doing conversation analysis* (2nd ed.). Sage.

Vickers, C. H., & Goble, R. (2018). Politeness and prosody in the co-construction of medical provider persona styles and patient relationships. *Journal of Applied Linguistics and Professional Practice, 11*(2), 202–226.

Wodak, R., & Meyer, M. (2009). *Methods of critical discourse analysis* (2nd ed.). Sage.

Wray, A., & Bloomer, A. (2012). *Projects in linguistics and language studies* (3rd ed.). Routledge.

Zayts, O., & Schnurr, S. (2014). More than 'information provider' and 'counselor': Constructing and negotiating roles and identities of nurses in genetic counseling sessions. *Journal of Sociolinguistics, 18*(3), 345–369.

3

ETHICS IN HEALTH AND LANGUAGE RESEARCH

3.1 Introduction

In the previous chapter, we looked at how you might plan a small research project and the methods you could employ. But what other considerations are important in designing a project? One area that will inform your project planning is 'research ethics'. Imagine, for example, you are writing a proposal for a small piece of independent research for your dissertation. You are interested in finding out about people's concerns in relation to a particular health issue, such as attitudes to vaccines, a topic touched on in the case study in Chapter 11. You are planning to interview a few people in a group and also to look at comments people have posted in response to news articles on the topic. At these preparatory stages, some of the practical questions you might be thinking about are:

- How can I make sure my group participants have enough information about why I want to speak to them?
- How can I ensure that people feel comfortable talking to me about personal subjects, including their health?
- Should I treat information from the people I interview differently to the people whose online comments I collect?
- How will I make sure my group participants (as well as the people who posted comments online) are not embarrassed if I publish my research, where others may be able to read about them?
- How will I safely store my recordings/downloads/transcripts of what people say on this topic?

These are questions that need to be considered when planning research and largely fall under 'research ethics' – at its simplest, the practices and behaviours one might

DOI: 10.4324/9781003020417-4

consider to be right or wrong during the research process. Researchers have a responsibility to avoid causing harm to people in a project, particularly where using material (or 'data') those people have provided. With origins in the field of 'biomedical sciences' (biologically and medically related disciplines), discussion of research ethics has become increasingly prominent in the Social Sciences and Applied Linguistics. In these contexts, 'data' tends to mean something different and often refers to texts people produce. The 'harm' this data can cause can be difficult to assess but information related to people's health – even in the form of descriptions of how they feel – can be highly sensitive. As we will explore, this risk of 'harm' could mean causing distress, damaging people's social relationships, or reducing their willingness to access healthcare services. Researchers need to think about whether their research poses risks, what they might do to mitigate these and, in turn, what benefits doing the research might have.

Research ethics can feel like a daunting area and the purpose of this chapter is not to put you off your chosen project but to get you to think through ethical issues right from the start. We cover two key areas: ethical *principles* for research and the more *procedural* aspects of research ethics applications. We start with some general guidance and principles (section 3.2) and then consider types of data and participants that might be employed (section 3.3), such as with:

- Public domain material;
- User-generated content online;
- Research interviews and focus groups;
- Fieldwork, observational and recorded data from healthcare settings;
- Secondary datasets.

The chapter goes on to address practicalities of keeping data confidential and non-identifiable (section 3.4) as well as potential risks to the researcher (section 3.5). Inevitably, there is much more to say about using sensitive or *higher* risk data than there is for more low-risk projects and so not everything will be relevant to your study. It may be that, having read this chapter and consulted with a supervisor, you are able to identify the risk of harm as being low for your particular study and that therefore not all of the advice will apply.

Nevertheless, it is crucial to think about these issues early on, as well as to check your university's procedural requirements. In some circumstances, you may need to apply for formal ethical approval from your university, perhaps from a tutor or a research ethics committee, before you can commence work. We offer some practical advice on this (section 3.6), focusing largely on the UK context, but you will need to check the requirements for your own university and jurisdiction – particularly since this will not apply to every project.

3.2 Ethical principles and considerations

What principles can you apply to ensure that research is ethical? There are some well-known frameworks outlining core ethical ideas for conducting research, many of which were established in biomedical contexts, such as the Declaration of Helsinki (World Medical Association, 2001) and the Belmont Report (1979). The 'Belmont Principles', which were drawn up to protect people in healthcare research after some problematic studies, are some of the most widely used and include:

- *Beneficence* (ensuring the wellbeing of participants) and *Non-maleficence* (avoiding causing harm to them);
- *Respect for individuals* (recognizing their autonomy, ensuring informed consent to the research and providing additional protections for those who might be vulnerable);
- *Justice* (treating people equitably and keeping in mind who should benefit most from the research).

(Beauchamp & Childress, 2001)

These broad principles around avoiding harm, treating people respectfully and striving for something beneficial from research are hard to disagree with. As outlined in the Introduction, the potential for harm is broad ranging, and is defined as, 'risks of psychological harm, physical harm, legal harm, social harm and economic harm' (Belmont Report, 1979, Part C). Psychological harm might include aspects such as the potential to cause distress by raising upsetting topics. Social harm might mean causing people embarrassment or difficulty within their communities or workplaces through the revelation of private information. Economic harm might be the costs involved for participants, for example if they have to travel to interviews or cover childcare costs. These are all effects that research in the social sciences can have.

While generally applicable, these broad principles can also make for a difficult 'fit' in the social sciences (Agar, 1996; Murphy & Dingwall, 2001). Consulting more subject-specific or regional codes, which can advise on particular approaches, is helpful for thinking through risks. For example,

- UK – ESRC's *Framework for research ethics* in the UK (ESRC, 2015) https://www.ukri.org/councils/esrc/guidance-for-applicants/research-ethics -guidance/framework-for-research-ethics/;
- UK – The British Association for Applied Linguistics, *Recommendations on Good Practice in Applied Linguistics* (2021) (also adopted by the International Association of Applied Linguistics) – henceforth referred to as the 'BAAL *Recommendations*';
- USA – The Linguistics Society of America – www.linguisticsociety.org/ resource/ethics;
- AoIR – Internet Research: Ethical Guidelines 3.0: https://aoir.org/reports/ ethics3.pdf, Franzke et al. (2020), henceforth referred to as AoIR Guidelines (2020).

We will refer to some of these documents when addressing specific types of data below. Ultimately though, no code can ever be comprehensive – the BAAL

Recommendations in fact acknowledge the need to assess ethics on a case-by-case basis. You will probably have to make some decisions during a project that are specific to your particular topic and data.

3.2.1 Research relationships – 'Subjects', 'respondents', 'informants', or 'participants'?

Before we address types of data, it is worth thinking about how to describe the people whose language we research. In the example in the Introduction, we asked if the data from the people interviewed about a healthcare topic should be treated differently to those whose online comments are collected. Are they 'subjects', 'respondents', 'informants', or 'participants'? In part, different relationships and responsibilities to people become denoted through the terms used to describe them, which vary between methods. The term 'subjects' is sometimes used in experimental research methods and can suggest a one-sided relationship, but can also be a more general term to describe any individual studied within the research (the term used by the Belmont Report in describing 'human subjects' research). 'Respondents' can be used in studies that make use of surveys, interviews, or focus groups – all typically settings where the researcher is asking questions of people, such as the example of interviews on a healthcare topic. 'Informants' is a term that has been used in anthropology and ethnography, where the researcher is learning about the practices and culture of a particular group or community. Finally, the term 'participant', which is perhaps most favoured in research ethics frameworks, implies a more active role for the people involved – more than simply 'subjects' to be protected. This active involvement might be particularly important in health, where the researcher is seeking to access lived experiences of other people. However, though favoured, the term 'participant' can be tricky if you are collecting data where there is no feasible way to directly involve people, particularly online settings, such as the example of collecting comments from a news article (see section 3.3.2). The AoIR (2020) guidelines use various terms, including 'authors' and 'subjects' to describe people whose online texts researchers collect. There are divided opinions on which terms are 'better' but, although you may have some restrictions from the ethics framework you work within, where possible it is good to use terms that actually reflect your research relationships.

3.3 Types of research participants and data

3.3.1 Research with media and public domain material

There is a wide variety of material available through television, radio, and news media, published literature, as well as public health campaigns, that can be fruitful for research on health communication. This material in the 'public domain' can often be easily accessed for research, without a great deal of ethical risk. In the UK for example, communications from public health campaigns by

the government or the National Health Service (NHS) can generally be analysed for research purposes without significant copyright or ethical restrictions.
Chapter 4 of this volume uses material from the UK's Covid-19 health campaigns in this way and there are examples of literary representations of illness in
Chapter 5. Although the risks of causing harm to people with these types of data
are lower, that does not mean there are no ethical considerations and you still
need to think about how you treat such material. In an important example from
literary analysis in this book (Chapter 5), authors Demjén and Semino (2015,
2021) outline their stylistic analysis of the book *Henry's Demons* (Cockburn &
Cockburn, 2011), which gives a first-hand account of experiences of schizophrenia. Demjén and Semino were mindful of the potential consequences in how
they represented Henry's perspective on schizophrenia, respecting his 'expertise through experience' as well as his view that his experiences were not a
'symptom' of a mental illness (section 5.3.1). The overarching ethical principle of
respect for people, outlined in 3.2 above, certainly extends to texts in the public
domain such as this and, since material is likely to be widely available and near
impossible to anonymize, it may require particular care and respectful analysis.

Depending on your institution, you may be able to use these types of public
domain material without an ethics application (a process described in section 3.6)
but you will need to check. If you plan to publish your research you may also
need to check copyright restrictions. Often, a proportion of published or broadcast material can be used and published as part of an academic analysis – a principle known as 'fair dealing' in the UK – but this is something you need to
confirm for your chosen data and local context. You can also check copyright
licences (most Creative Commons licensing, for example, allows material to be
reused in published research) and, if necessary, seek rights permissions from the
original publisher. Where you encounter difficulties, there are also other solutions: for the study highlighted in Chapter 9, Harvey (2013) managed copyright
concerns by commissioning outline images for some of the website material he
analysed, allowing him to show sufficient detail to evidence his findings.

3.3.2 *Research with user-generated online content*

An area which has seen rapid expansion in linguistic data on health is the wide
variety of 'new media' content produced through the internet and digital technologies. These environments have provided a means for people to rapidly share
and consume information and perspectives about health, including seeking advice
from professionals (Chapter 7) and in online health communities (Chapter 8).
Data from these online contexts presents important research avenues for linguists. For example, we introduced the idea above of collecting online comments
from news articles about vaccination. Unlike interviews, it would be hard to ask
the authors of such comments for permission to use their words in research. This
type of 'user-generated' content (material that has been posted by people using
online platforms, such as comments, discussion forums, blogs, photo, and video

sharing through social media) can present ethical challenges. Some complexities are outlined below to get you thinking about your research, but do keep in mind throughout that collecting texts from online settings can, by and large, be a fruitful and practical source of data.

Although user-generated content might be available in the public domain, the authors themselves may not always see their material as 'public'. Distinct social contexts and the boundaries between public and private are seen to have collapsed for online texts (boyd, 2011: 45), making intended audiences ambiguous. There is evidence to suggest that some users perceive their interactions within an online group to have a degree of privacy, even if the group is an open one (Frankel & Siang, 1999). If this is the case, then there is perhaps the potential to cause some degree of social or psychological harm by analyzing and publishing people's written material in a different, i.e. research, context that they are unlikely to have anticipated. It might feel like a violation for the authors, potentially reducing their willingness to engage further in those contexts or damaging their existing relationships. This risks reducing the benefits people gain from communicating with others in online settings. If you are using texts from such online settings, you may want to assess people's likely expectation of privacy according to:

- whether or not the forum or website requires a login to access (Elm, 2009);
- whether there are a large number of members, which might suggest contributions are understood as being more 'public' (Eysenbach & Till, 2001);
- whether 'to take into account not just the affordances of a site, but the extent to which the participants who are authoring social media materials indicate that their writing is publicly available', such as how users address their messages to others (Page et al., 2014: 67). A blog, for example, might be much more open in who it directly addresses than an illness support group;
- whether the website terms and conditions refer to the use of posted material in research.

Some online texts, such as comments on news articles, are generally pseudo-anonymous and by definition very public in nature, meaning they can be used with low ethical risk (Collins, 2019). It is generally advisable to use 'openly' available material such as this but, if a decision is made that there is a degree of 'privacy' to the online texts, you may want to consider ways to get permission from the authors (outlined further in section 3.6.1).

This public/private distinction is an issue Mackenzie (2017) grapples with, describing a shift in her understanding of an online Mumsnet discussion forum from a public to a more private setting as she herself shifted to an 'observer-as-participant'. This co-participation in the group led Mackenzie to make an ethical decision to gain users' explicit consent for the research. In more 'private' online contexts or where participant observation is a core part of the methodology, consent from individuals is likely to be important. In the example of digital ethnography outlined in Chapter 8, Koteyko and Hunt (2016) become online participant observers in analyzing Facebook profiles depicting identities around diabetes. The research was only possible by getting consent directly from all the people involved. It also meant excluding certain environments, such as private messaging and closed groups, from the immediate field of study (p. 61). In other settings, such co-participation may not always be practical or even ethical. For example, Hunt and Brookes (2020) conduct research on the language of online health communities on the topics of depression, anorexia and diabulimia. They discuss how it would have been impractical at this corpus scale to become active 'participant observers' in these mental health fora but also potentially disingenuous since the researchers did not have direct experience of the conditions they were interested in (pp. 71–75).

For some types of user-content, such as health advice columns that people send queries to, the websites themselves may have gained blanket permission for use of the material in research. This was the case for the Teenage Health Freak (Mullany et al., 2015) and the 'Lucy Answers' website data (Locher, 2006) described in Chapter 7. While it may not be necessary (or possible) to ask individual users for further permission for use this material, permission may still need to be given by the website (as was the case for Teenage Health Freak) and it will be important to consider how the anonymity of the texts' authors can continue to be maintained in your analysis and quotes (see section 3.4).

Decisions about the public/private nature of online data and who, if anyone, you need to seek permission from are complex and context-dependent. You should draw on the guidance at your own institution as well as documents such as the AoIR guidelines (2020) and the recent version of the BAAL *Recommendations* (2021) to help with your decisions. However, do keep in mind that in general, for many studies of online data that draw on publicly available and often anonymous material, the ethical risks are limited.

3.3.3 *Research interviews and focus groups*

A source of data suggested in the Introduction was interviewing people about a particular health topic such as vaccines. Research interviews are used for a variety of methodologies and can be a manageable option for short studies. They usually involve the researcher posing a series of questions to a 'respondent' or 'participant'. They can be 'structured', where the researcher will ask a list of standardized questions, 'semi-structured', or 'unstructured', which become more like guided conversations. 'Focus groups' are a related form, sometimes treated as 'group interviews', where the same questions can be posed to a number of respondents at the same time.

Here there is a very clear ethical requirement to gain people's consent to take part (the procedural requirements for which are outlined further in section 3.6.1). In addition, there are some general ethical considerations for all forms of interviews. Firstly, while interviews can be a good setting in which to gain insight into sensitive health topics and personal experiences, they can risk causing distress to participants if topics are particularly upsetting to them. Imagine for example, if someone has to describe losing a relative to Covid-19 in an interview on attitudes to vaccines. To conduct an interview ethically, you should ideally think about whether the topics you raise have the potential to cause distress and, if so, how you might warn people. You should also think about what you could do in these circumstances, such as turning off a recording device, checking with the participant if they are happy to continue and, in some instances, sensitively pointing them to where they can seek support (see Draucker et al., 2009 for further discussion).

It is also possible that respondents might reveal details about others that could cause offence or embarrassment within their own community and you will need to think about how details can be sufficiently obscured to avoid this, particularly if you later want to publish your work (see section 3.4). For linguistic research, it is likely you will want to record and transcribe the interviews, rather than simply take notes. You will need to think about how you will safely store the recordings and, where necessary, anonymize them and the details they contain. It may not be enough simply to remove people's names and locations but other details, such as descriptions of colleagues, might also need to be obscured. The BAAL *Recommendations* (2021) highlight how it can also be good practice to send respondents the transcripts of the interviews, to check if they are comfortable with what has been said or if there is anything they would wish to be removed.

For a variety of reasons (including the changes during the Covid-19 pandemic), you might choose to conduct interviews remotely, either over the phone or via video conferencing tools. There are considerations here in terms of the technological literacy of participants and what they will feel comfortable using. Not only will you need a space from which to conduct these interviews as the researcher, you will also need to think about the fact that it can be harder for participants to find a quiet and private setting. It can also be harder in a remote interview to tell when a participant is distressed and you could consider having 'check points' to see if participants are still happy to continue.

If people are giving up their time for research interviews, it can be helpful to compensate them, although you would not ordinarily be expected to do this for a short student project. You can get ethical guidance more specifically related to interviews in the UK context from the Oral History Society (www.ohs.org .uk/legal-and-ethical-advice/) and the British Psychological Society (www.bps .org.uk/guideline/bps-practice-guidelines-2017-0). There are also important considerations around respondents whose first language is different to yours (see section 3.6.3) and researcher safety when conducting interviews (see section 3.5).

3.3.4 Fieldwork, observational, and recorded data from healthcare settings

'Fieldwork' is where a researcher goes into a setting to observe or record data about people and their interactions, as they occur in situ (see Chapter 6). It can also incorporate types of online, digital ethnography (as in Chapter 8). Research fieldwork will usually involve coming into contact with a number of people and you will need to ensure you maintain respectful relationships with all of them. Such research is perhaps only feasible for projects where you have an extended amount of time available but can be enormously rewarding and result in rich data, as you become familiar with the people and groups you are observing. It can, though, be quite unpredictable – unexpected things happen and you might need to make ethical decisions in situ, such as quickly stopping a recording during a medical emergency or perhaps reminding participants about your role as a researcher if they begin to treat you as a friend. These have been described as 'ethically important moments' that can arise during a project (Guillemin & Gillam, 2004) and involve thinking about 'ethics in practice' (beyond the more regulatory aspect of ethics applications). If you plan to do fieldwork, you will almost certainly need to gain formal ethical approval, outlined further in section 3.6. Part of this will involve gaining the consent of the people you observe, also described in 3.6.1. You may also therefore need to consider your institution's guidance on mitigating risks during fieldwork or working 'off-site'. These also include risks to you as a researcher (for more on this, see section 3.5)

3.3.5 Secondary data

'Secondary data' is material that has already been collected by another researcher for a project and then made available to be reused for new projects and research questions. It can be a good alternative to collecting entirely new ('primary') data for a small-scale research project. There are some great openly available language datasets that may be appropriate to use in a project on health communication, such as the medical consultations contained within the original spoken British National Corpus (www.natcorp.ox.ac.uk/). Online datasets are also sometimes created by and shared between researchers: the #ReframeCovid database, discussed in Chapter 10, is an open collection of metaphors for the Covid-19 pandemic, as alternatives to the dominant 'war' framing (https://sites.google.com /view/reframecovid/initiative). For this, researchers sent examples, including entries in multiple languages, which were then published in an open source document for anyone to use. Since these examples come from openly available, public documents there are low risks of harm to particular people and the ethical considerations are minimal, but you will still want to check with a tutor or supervisor and treat the material respectfully.

It is always worth looking at what may be available through 'data repositories', which hold collections of data specifically for secondary use in research. Material from publicly funded research will often be made available through digital repositories, such as the UK Data Service (https://ukdataservice.ac.uk/). In healthcare, the sharing of data is complex since information about people's health rightly holds protections. However, some types of data are increasingly becoming available through repositories, often with some degree of restriction or access conditions. Databases of written patient records are beginning to emerge (e.g. the Clinical Records Interactive Search 'CRIS' at the Maudsley Hospital: www.maudsleybrc.nihr.ac.uk/facilities/clinical-record-interactive -search-cris/), which may have scope for use in linguistic research. There are also datasets with a greater social science focus, such as the 'One in a Million' collection of videoed GP consultations: (www.bristol.ac.uk/primaryhealthcare /researchthemes/one-in-a-million/). Secondary datasets such as these usually require the researcher to complete an access application and often gain ethical approval, which can take some time, so are not always an 'easy' option for short term projects. Nevertheless, they can be valuable for accessing large-scale data in a PhD and other Postgraduate research that would otherwise be infeasible for a lone researcher.

3.4 Anonymizing data

Some of the risks outlined above involve potential embarrassment to research participants in making their language data, personal details or views on health topics known publicly or to their friends, family, and colleagues. Imagine, for example, from the study proposed in the Introduction above, that a healthcare professional expresses a personal view about vaccinations that their colleagues would likely disagree with. Revealing this could cause that person difficulties in their job. Some of these risks can be mitigated through anonymizing research data.

If your data come from publicly available broadcast media, then in general you will not need to anonymize but if you have recorded or collected data more privately then it is best practice to obscure participants' identities and to tell them you will do so. If you are planning to publish your work these issues become even more acute. Murphy and Dingwall (2001) highlight that linguistic researchers may need to recognize the point of publication as a critical moment in the potential to cause harm, since it is at this point that private information revealed during the research process might become recognizable to others, perhaps with risks of social harm within people's communities.

There are reasonable steps the researcher can take to ensure that identities of participants are protected as far as possible. This usually means changing names and locations mentioned, often providing pseudonyms instead. Antaki (2002) gives a useful 'ten guidelines' on anonymizing spoken data. However, anonymization does not always prevent all risk of identification: Deborah Cameron (2001: 23) recounts a story of how she happened to be able to identify a woman she had once met in New York just from the transcripts in a journal article. If anonymity is crucially important, you could consider using short quotes from your data, to prevent identification from a longer string of details revealed by extended extracts. Textual data can sometimes make complete anonymization hard in linguistics and if you are consenting participants (see 3.6.1) you will need to be clear about the extent of anonymization you can realistically achieve.

The public/private nature of online content will be a particularly important consideration in terms of rendering people identifiable. While it might be possible to change names and identifying details in the quotes you use, online texts have the unique risk of being easily searchable so that the original text can be found. Where necessary, it might be possible to protect the privacy of user-generated data through giving pseudonyms and drawing on material not indexed through search engines (so that any published quotes are not easily retrievable through an online search). You also need to check the terms and conditions of the site that hosts the original content. Twitter, for example, stated, at the time of writing, that the username must be displayed and that the text must not be modified when giving quotes.

Having said all that, texts and their authors becoming identifiable might not always present a high risk of harm, particularly where posts are very public and seen as such by the authors. Some have questioned whether there are instances in which naming identifiable participants might in fact be more ethical, as long as the research is conducted respectfully (Moore, 2012). Often authors themselves will also have already obscured their identities online. Comments on news articles, for example, are usually posted under people's self-chosen pseudonyms, so searching for a quote may not risk easy identification with their real identities (although even this needs caution – the AoIR 2020 guidelines highlight the release of supposedly anonymized dating profiles that were easily re-linked to people (p. 20)). Williams et al. (2017) provide a useful decision tree for thinking through the quotation of tweets in publications that could also be applied to online data more generally. The decision around identification and anonymization will be something you need to weigh up carefully for online data, thinking through the risks involved, guidance in documents such as AoIR (2020) and any advice from your tutor or university.

3.5 Risks to the researcher

So far we have discussed ethical principles largely in terms of protecting participants. While this is the chief concern of research ethics and should certainly be a key focus, an aspect that has increasingly been considered as an ethical issue is the potential for harm to researchers themselves. There are recognized risks around researcher safety, particularly where you might be conducting interviews or fieldwork outside of university premises. It can be appropriate to take a chaperone if interviewing people away from public spaces and you should always let someone know where you are planning to go. Though perhaps unlikely in healthcare research, if you are doing online research in hostile contexts, there are suggestions in the AoIR guidelines (2020) about protecting your own identity.

But researcher wellbeing encompasses more than these overt risks of harm – it also covers the potential for research to cause psychological harm, particularly if researchers are looking at sensitive or emotionally distressing topics. At some point during our lives, most of us will be impacted by health difficulties, whether that be ourselves or our friends and family, and these experiences may impact the way in which research on this topic affects us. Sometimes, working with data can affect a researcher in a way that they were not expecting, such as where they hear or read about someone else's upsetting experience, whether or not this is coloured by their own experiences. The emotional toll of distressing research should not be overlooked (Rüdiger & Dayter, 2017) and this issue is now a topic in its own right in the revised BAAL *Recommendations* (2021).

Being affected by data you spend long periods analyzing is normal and does not necessarily mean that you are not maintaining sufficient distance between yourself and your project. It can be helpful to think about how you might plan for research that is potentially primed to cause distress. Before selecting a topic and data source, it is worth thinking about whether you actually feel this is something you will be able to study and analyze for long periods of time. Potentially distressing areas do not need to be avoided altogether, though, and there are techniques you can use to help manage difficulties. For example, you can plan to only work on the data during specific periods of time and, where possible, in a separate space to where you sleep or spend time relaxing. This helps to give a good cut off point for thinking about the data. Talking about your research with fellow students or a supervisor can also help to manage the emotional toll of research.

3.6 Regulatory ethics and applications

In many countries and institutions research that involves 'human subjects' (which, as we have seen, can include language produced *by* or *about* people) requires an application for ethical approval. How you do this will vary according to the university, institution or jurisdiction you are in. As a student, you may need to submit a form outlining your project to your module leader or supervisor. For larger projects or as an independent researcher, you may need to submit a full application to a Research Ethics Committee (REC) or Institutional Review Board (IRB). It is important to plan well ahead for this. If you are unsure about the process required, seek advice from a supervisor or tutor at an early stage to ensure that you do not encounter problems later down the line. If you do need to complete an application, it should detail your research objectives, design and the data you plan to collect, identifying potential issues and how you plan to mitigate these. These risks encompass the potential for psychological, social or economic harm for people who participate, outlined in section 3.2, as well as risks to you, the researcher, as discussed in section 3.5.

Filling out ethics documentation can feel hard but it is worth treating it as more than a tick box exercise and use the process to reflect on your research design and the principles outlined in the first part of this chapter. Although the ethics application is undoubtedly a gate-keeping stage, it is also an opportunity to gain feedback about how best to conduct your project, highlighting aspects that you may not have thought about, as the case study in Chapter 10 of this book highlights. Questions on the application form are likely to ask you about ethical issues that may arise from the research but no ethics committee will expect you to remove risks altogether – it is how you manage and minimize these that is important, as well as weighing this against the benefits of the research. For example, if you plan to interview people about attitudes to vaccines you might identify some risk of embarrassment if their views were to become known to their friends and family and so could plan to mitigate these risks through anonymizing your data, outlining the overall benefits for better knowledge in this area. You will find further guidance in the earlier parts of this chapter.

If your application is going to a research ethics committee, keep in mind that this may consist of people who do not specialize in your methodology or even your field, so you need to explain your research design in a way that can be understood by non-experts. It is rare for an ethics application to be rejected but there might be queries or requests for changes to your research design that you need to respond to. Often suggested changes can be useful but you may feel some are inappropriate. In these instances it is certainly possible to counter the suggestions with an explanation about methods or justification as to how the benefits of your research outweigh the anticipated risks – an example of this is given in Chapter 10 on a project with healthcare professionals in 'Schwartz Center Rounds', justifying the data collection from real-life contexts.

Finally, it is worth noting that some projects in healthcare can constitute a 'special case' in many countries and, unlike other fields, may require an application through a specially designed or nationally agreed application process, such as to a medical research ethics committee. In the UK, for example, it can sometimes be necessary to apply to an NHS research ethics committee. By no means does this cover all research in healthcare but, if you are unsure, this is something you will need to gain specific advice about from your supervisor or your research organization.

3.6.1 Informed consent with participants

If you plan on creating 'primary data', such as conducting interviews or recording people talking, you will need to gain informed consent from participants. There may also be contexts in which you collect existing material but still make the ethical decision to consent people (such as collecting data from some online contexts, described in section 3.1.1). Gaining consent of course means asking people if they are happy to be included in your study and, to be meaningful, consent should be given freely with the option to be withdrawn. This respects people's rights to autonomy, outlined in section 3.2, ensuring that people do not feel coerced into participating, particularly where there is a power asymmetry. For example, a youth group leader gaining consent from young people in their group to be part of a study would need to ensure that they do not feel obligated to participate and that this has no bearing on their relationships within the setting. Similarly, consenting patients for a study requires that this will have no perceived detrimental effect on accessing care.

In terms of regulatory requirements, consenting people usually involves creating a 'Participant Information Sheet' (PIS) and corresponding 'Consent Form' to give to potential participants. The PIS provides written information about the project, to help people to decide whether they want to take part. The particular format and information required will be specified at your university, but it usually needs to include the following information:

- the title of the project;
- the name and contact details of the researcher;
- an explanation of the project in plain language;
- a summary of the risks and benefits of taking part;
- an invitation to the participant to take part and explanation of why they have been invited;
- assurance that participation is voluntary and details of how they can withdraw;
- an explanation of what will happen to participants' data, including whether their data may be published and reused in other contexts;
- confirmation that the project has received ethical approval (and usually contact details of the institution and details for further queries/concerns/complaints);
- a 'thank you' to the participant for their time.

The accompanying consent form is what the participant then signs, following their decision to participate. Again, you will need to check the guidance and templates used by your own institution but consent forms usually include terms like the following:

- I have read and understood the information in the Participant Information Sheet which I have been given to read and a copy to keep;
- I have been given the opportunity to ask questions about the study;
- I have had my questions answered satisfactorily by the research team;
- I understand that my data will be stored securely and confidentially, and will be anonymized as quickly as possible;
- I agree that my anonymized data may be used in reports and outcomes from the project;
- I understand that my participation is voluntary and that I am free to withdraw at any time until the data has been anonymized, without the need to give a reason.

It is important to include as much relevant information as you can about the study, to enable people to exercise their right to make an informed decision. Nevertheless, documents must also not be so long that the participant is unlikely to be able to read them in the time available, particularly if you are consenting people 'on site'. As the researcher, you need to be available to explain the forms and answer further questions, whether that be in person or remotely. It may be that you receive questions or issues arise that you had not expected, and these are the kinds of moments that you need to carefully exercise your own ethical decision making to ensure you answer accurately. The UK data service provides further very detailed advice on putting together information sheets and consent forms (https://ukdataservice.ac.uk/media /622375/ukdamodelconsent.docx).

3.6.2 Vulnerable participants

If participants come from a vulnerable group, special care must be taken in relation to their consent and the conduct of the research to ensure their safety and wellbeing. This might include research with people who are not able to fully consent for themselves, such as children or those 'without capacity' (where you may also be required to gain consent from a third party, such as a parent or a patient's family member), or people who may be vulnerable within a particular context, such as survivors of trauma or people with serious health conditions. There is some useful guidance on working with vulnerable participants from UK Research and Innovation (www.ukri.org/councils/esrc/guidance-for-appli-cants/research-ethics-guidance/research-with-potentially-vulnerable-people/) as well as in the BAAL *Recommendations* (2021). You should be aware that consenting these groups of people is ethically complex and, in general, it is likely to be beyond the scope of a small study. If you are unsure if your participants are likely to be vulnerable, this is something you should check with a supervisor at an early stage of project planning, given the effect it will have on your research design and ethics.

3.6.3 Intercultural ethics

Regulatory processes for gaining ethical approval and consent from participants are, by and large, drawn from Western contexts. While information sheets and consent forms tend to adhere to a standard format, you may need to think about varying the way you consent participants in other settings. If you are researching in a multilingual setting, for example, documents may at least need to be available in more than one language for participants. The BAAL *Recommendations* (2021) also outline how recording oral consent may be more appropriate than written forms in some circumstances, particularly where literacy may be an issue, although this approach should be justified in your application for ethical approval.

   Copland and Creese (2015) address other issues around intercultural ethics, including situations in which the regulatory processes of signing consent forms can cause distrust and confusion, even being potentially damaging to participants (p. 185–6). Where participants are sought from different sociocultural groups, it is worth gaining some input from them on practices that might affect how a formal consent process is perceived and the best means of asking permission for the study.

3.6.4 Data protection laws

As a researcher, you will need to adhere to the data protection laws of your country or jurisdiction. Data protection is a legal matter, rather than a specifically ethical one, but some of the requirements are motivated by ethical considerations for people's privacy. Data protection laws might also have implications for keeping hold of participants' contact details, such as for sending research results at a later date or reconsenting for further reuse of the data, and you should ask for permission to store these. These matters are likely to be covered in your institution's general guidance and some advice on the UK context can also be found in the BAAL *Recommendations* (2021: section 2.5). If you are using secondary data (see 3.3.5), you may also need to fill out and agree data protection paperwork with the original data owners, providing assurances about how you will store and use the data. Your research office or data protection officer at your university should be able to assist with this.

3.7 Concluding remarks

This chapter has highlighted how research ethics, that is, the good practices for conducting research, especially when it involves people, is an important part of planning a project in language and health. Some linguistics projects in healthcare involve textual data that details sensitive information about people's experiences of and attitudes to health and therefore needs to be collected and treated with care. Some core principles for ethical research conduct are respect for people's *autonomy*, i.e. giving them the right to choose to take part in a study with full information on what it is about, as well as *beneficence*, *non-maleficence*, and *justice* in the way your research achieves benefits for and avoids harm to people. It is wise to consult some subject-specific guidance and think about the particular context you are researching when considering ethical issues that may come up. Keep in mind though that research ethics is important to think about for the life of a project – you might well encounter issues that you had not originally considered and need to make a decision about how best to manage these. Alongside these important principles and practices for research, we also outlined that some studies may entail *procedural* ethical requirements at your university, such as gaining approval from a supervisor or ethics committee. Early on in designing your study, check what the requirements are as one of your first tasks.

Further readings

British Association for Applied Linguistics (BAAL). (2021). *Recommendations on good practice in applied linguistics.* Retrieved from https://www.baal.org.uk/who-we-are/resources/

Bryman, A. (2021). *Social research methods* (6th ed.). OUP (see Chapter 6 on research ethics).

BSA. Ethical guidelines and collated resources for digital research. Retrieved from www .britsoc.co.uk/media/24309/bsa_statement_of_ethical_practice_annexe.pdf

Franzke, A. S., Bechmann, A., Zimmer, M., Ess, C., & the Association of Internet Researchers. (2020). *Internet research: Ethical guidelines 3.0.* Retrieved from https://aoir .org/reports/ethics3.pdf

References

Agar, M. (1996). *The professional stranger: An informal introduction to ethnography* (2nd ed.). Emerald Group Publishing Limited.

Antaki, C. (2002). An introductory tutorial in conversation analysis. Retrieved October 10, 2022, from http://ca-tutorials.lboro.ac.uk/sitemenu.htm

Beauchamp, T. L., & Childress, J. F. (2001). *Principles of biomedical ethics.* Oxford University Press.

Boyd, D. (2011). Social network sites as networked publics: Affordances, dynamics, and implications. In Z. Papacharissi (Ed.), *A networked self: Identity, community, and culture on social network sites* (pp. 39–58). Routledge.

British Association for Applied Linguistics (BAAL). (2021). *Recommendations on good practice in applied linguistics.* Retrieved from https://www.baal.org.uk/wp-content/ uploads/2021/03/BAAL-Good-Practice-Guidelines-2021.pdf

Cameron, D. (2001). *Working with spoken discourse.* Sage.

Cockburn, P., & Cockburn, H. (2011). *Henry's Demons living with schizophrenia: A father and son story.* Simon & Schuster.

Collins, L. (2019). *Corpus linguistics for online communication: A guide for research.* Routledge.

Copland, F., & Creese, A. (2015). *Linguistic ethnography: Collecting, analysing and presenting data.* Sage.

Demjén, Z., & Semino, E. (2015). Henry's voices: The representation of auditory verbal hallucinations in an autobiographical narrative. *BMJ Medical Humanities, 41*(1), 57–62.

Demjén, Z., & Semino, E. (2021). Stylistics: Mind style in an autobiographical account of schizophrenia. In G. Brookes & D. Hunt (Eds.), *Analysing health communication: Discourse approaches* (pp. 333–356). Palgrave.

Draucker, C. B., Martsolf, D. S., & Poole, C. (2009). Developing distress protocols for research on sensitive topics. *Archives of Psychiatric Nursing, 23*(5), 343–350.

ESRC. (2015). Economic and social research council – Research ethics framework. Retrieved from https://esrc.ukri.org/files/funding/guidance-for-applicants/esrc -framework-for-research-ethics-2015/

Elm, M. S. (2009). How do various notions of privacy influence decisions in qualitative Internet research? In A. Markham & N. Baym (Eds.), *Internet inquiry: Dialogue among researchers* (pp. 69–87). Sage.

Eysenbach, G., & Till, J. E. (2001). Ethical issues in qualitative research on internet communities. *BMJ: British Medical Journal, 323*(7321), 1103–1105.

Frankel, M. S., & Siang, S. (1999). *Ethical and legal aspects of human subjects research on the Internet. A report of a workshop June 10–11, 1999,* Washington, DC. Retrieved from https://www.aaas.org/sites/default/files/report2.pdf

Franzke, A. S., Bechmann, A., Zimmer, M., Ess, C., & the Association of Internet Researchers. (2020). *Internet research: Ethical guidelines 3.0.* Retrieved from https://aoir .org/reports/ethics3.pdf

Guillemin, M., & Gillam, L. (2004). Ethics, reflexivity, and "ethically important moments" in research. *Qualitative Inquiry*, *10*(2), 261–280. Retrieved from https://journals.sagepub.com/doi/abs/10.1177/1077800403262360

Harvey, K. (2013). Medicalisation, pharmaceutical promotion and the Internet: A critical multimodal discourse analysis of hair loss websites. *Social Semiotics*, *23*(5), 691–714. https://doi.org/10.1080/10350330.2013.777596

Hunt, D., & Brookes, G. (2020). *Corpus, discourse and mental health*. Bloomsbury Publishing.

Koteyko, N., & Hunt, D. (2016). Performing health identities on social media: An online observation of Facebook profiles. *Discourse, Context and Media*, *12*, 59–67.

Locher, M. (2006). *Advice online: Advice-giving in an American Internet health column*. John Benjamins.

Mackenzie, J. (2017). Identifying informational norms in Mumsnet Talk: A reflexive-linguistic approach to internet research ethics. *Applied Linguistics Review*, *8*(2–3), 293–314.

Moore, N. (2012). The politics and ethics of naming: Questioning anonymisation in (archival) research. *International Journal of Social Research Methodology*, *15*(4), 331–340.

Mullany, L., Smith, C., Harvey, K., & Adolphs, S. (2015). 'Am I anorexic?' weight, eating and discourses of the body in online adolescent health communication. *Communication and Medicine*, *12*(2–3), 211–223.

Murphy, E., & Dingwall, R. (2001). The ethics of ethnography. In P. Atkinson, A. Coffey, S. Delamont, J. Lofland & L. Lofland (Eds.), *Doing qualitative research in primary care: Multiple strategies* (pp. 221–238). Sage.

National Commission for the Protection of Human Subjects of Biomedical and Behavioral Research. (1979). *The Belmont report: Ethical principles and guidelines for the protection of human subjects of research*. U.S. Department of Health and Human Services. Retrieved from https://www.hhs.gov/ohrp/regulations-and-policy/belmont-report/read-the-belmont-report/index.html

Page, R., Barton, D., Lee, C., Unger, J. W., & Zappavigna, M. (2014). *Researching language and social media: A student guide*. London: Routledge.

Rüdiger, S., & Dayter, D. (2017). The ethics of researching unlikeable subjects. *Applied Linguistics Review*, *8*(2–3), 251–269.

Williams, M., Burnap, P., & Sloan, L. (2017). Towards an ethical framework for publishing Twitter data in social research: Taking into account users' views, online context and algorithmic estimation. *Sociology*, *51*(6), 1149–1168.

World Medical Association. (2001). Declaration of Helsinki. Ethical principles for medical research involving human subjects. *Bulletin of the World Health Organization*, *79*(4), 373–374. Retrieved from https://apps.who.int/iris/handle/10665/26831

PART II

Investigating language and health

4

AGENCY, RESPONSIBILITY, AND RISK IN PUBLIC HEALTH COMMUNICATION

4.1 Introduction

The first part of the 21st century saw multiple serious disease outbreaks concentrated in different parts of the world: SARS in South East Asia, MERS in the Middle East, Ebola in West Africa, Zika in South America, and Covid-19 around the globe. Like many countries around the world, the United Kingdom experienced the start of the Covid-19 epidemic in early 2020. National governments responded to this public health crisis in different ways. South Korea, New Zealand, Vietnam, Senegal, and others opted for a so-called 'elimination' strategy (getting rid of the virus in the community completely), while most of Europe adopted a 'suppression' strategy (reducing the number of cases at any one time), which was often referred to as 'flattening the curve'. The United Kingdom was among those seen by some commentators as not taking decisive action fast enough, but it eventually moved towards a version of flattening the curve. At the time, with few effective treatments for Covid-19, and no vaccine yet available, behaviour change was the only way to achieve this suppression: the government had to tell people what to do and what not to do. In such situations, effective communication often means simple messaging and clarity on what behaviours need to change (Fishbein & Ajzen, 2010), communicated in a way that is most likely to encourage communities to comply.

At the end of March 2020, a seven-week lockdown began in the United Kingdom where people were told to stay at home, not go outside except for essential shopping and an hour of exercise per day. This message was distilled to 'Stay at home. Protect the NHS. Save lives'. as in Figure 4.1.

This slogan was set against a yellow background framed by red diagonal 'warning' stripes (Figure 4.1). In May 2020, when the first lockdown in the United Kingdom ended and restrictions were eased, the government changed its message

DOI: 10.4324/9781003020417-6

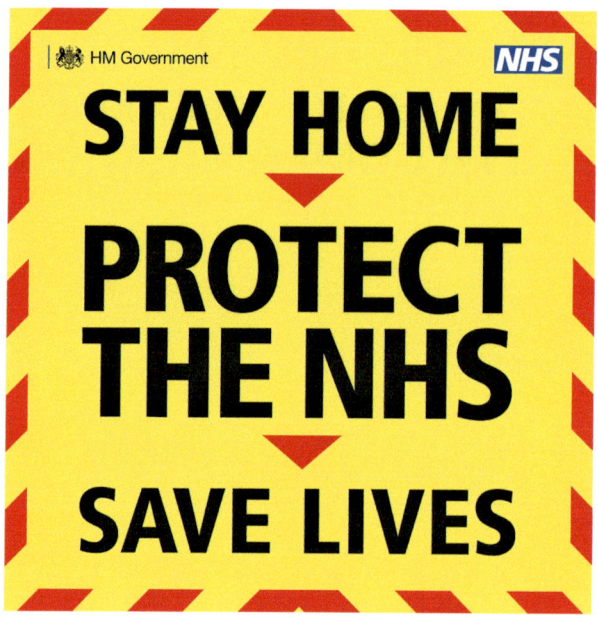

FIGURE 4.1 Stay at home. Protect the NHS. Save lives

both in colour scheme and in wording (Figure 4.2). The new slogan was no longer 'Stay at home' but 'Stay Alert'. You didn't need to 'Protect the NHS', you just had to 'Control the Virus', though you still had to 'Save Lives' (Figure 4.2).

All of this was now presented on a slightly brighter yellow background and with green warning stripes to frame it. Jones (2021) argues that, while decisions about layout and colour and font may seem trivial, they actually have a considerable impact on how effective particular messages are at mobilizing the public to act.

The new message generated a lot of critical commentary from the press and the public, especially on social media. One example of this debate, focusing on the verbal content of the message, occurred on the professional social networking site LinkedIn, initiated by branding and verbal identity consultant Chris West. In a brief video, West explained that his first impression of the new message was not that great, but he then changed his mind. He argued that 'Stay Alert' asks people to take direct action; it gives people something to do. At the same time, it doesn't give people everything; it doesn't tell people *how* to stay alert. While such ambiguity has disadvantages, it can also leave room for people to fill in the gap, which can increase engagement with the message. West invited his contacts on LinkedIn to provide their own views. Figure 4.3 shows excerpts from some of the responses.

These reactions illustrate some of the factors that can influence how a particular message is received. Much of the discussion focused on whether the message

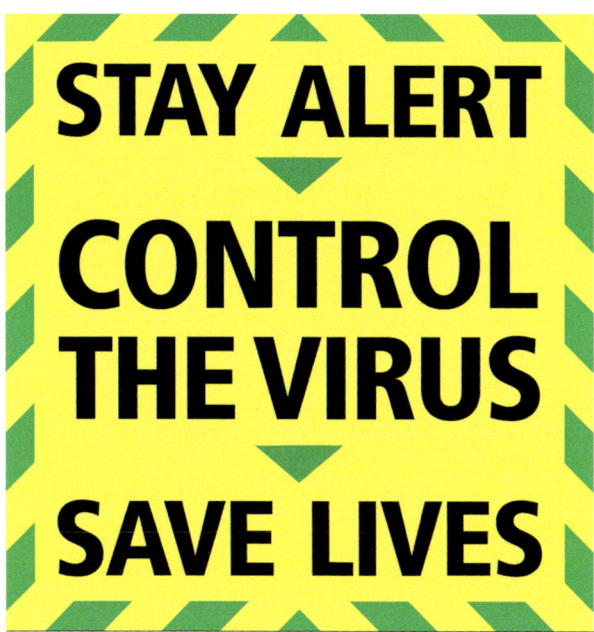

FIGURE 4.2   Stay alert. Control the virus. Save lives

was clear and effective, and more precisely 'what was it effective at'? People had different interpretations about what the motivation behind this new message was, and these tended to be linked to their attitudes to, and trust in the UK government, which was the source of the message. This nicely illustrates one complexity of public health communication: the effect of a public health message, particularly in the sense of compliance, is intricately connected with the level of trust people have in the source of the message otherwise (Wright et al., 2022, Sridhar, 2022). Another aspect of the message that influenced interpretations was the context in which it appeared. Some felt that you couldn't discuss this message on its own; you had to also consider all the political and communicative situations and controversies that had preceded it. These are the kinds of issues that are often of great concern to an approach in Linguistics called Critical Discourse Analysis (CDA).

CDA is an approach to the study of language and discourse in society, providing a 'theoretical perspective on language and more generally semiosis (including visual language, body language, and so on) … Which gives rise to ways of analysing language or semiosis within broader analyses of the social process' (Fairclough, 2001: 121). Simply put, CDA uses multiple methods or tools of analysis and focuses on how language reflects and maintains hierarchies and inequalities in the social world. So, in the assumptions that we make about why something is being communicated to us – why are we being asked to stay alert

> ...The new one IMO [in my opinion] completely fails to address me as an individual or link to a specific outcome. They had to go on to clarify what 'stay alert' could mean... (Kevin McLean)

> ...I do feel that instructing us simply to adopt a state of mind is a bit flabby right now. 'Stay Apart' (or similar) would have moved us on from 'Stay Home' and given people a degree of agency, but would still offer clear instruction... (Gill Ereaut)

> ... I think the success of any messaging is embedded in a broader (and historical) context – and I don't think the UK govt are in sufficient credit, in terms of how they have handled comms to date, to be given the benefit of the doubt!! (Emmet Ó Briain)

> ...the key to controlling the virus is through rigorous testing and tracking – something the Government has failed to master [...] Short of keeping us in permanent lockdown, how can they evolve the message to get round this problem? I know, shift responsibility onto the British public instead by suggesting that it is our success or failure at "staying alert" (whatever that means) that will control the virus... (Kate Miller)

FIGURE 4.3 Excerpts of responses on LinkedIn

rather than stay at home? Why are *we* being asked to control the virus? Is that a reasonable distribution of responsibility (and potentially blame if actions fail)? – and, in questioning those assumptions, we are trying to understand what hierarchies, equalities, and power dynamics are at play in any particular advice being given. We summarize examples of the types of studies that can be conducted under the umbrella of CDA in sections 4.3.1 and 4.3.2.

The change in colour scheme was another aspect of the two public health messages in Figure 4.1 and Figure 4.2 that drew critique. While visually the two messages are reasonably simple, the change from the first to the second was significant. According to ISO standard 3864-1:2011 – an internationally agreed standard for safety signs in public areas – red should be used for warnings, while green should be used for signs that signal safety, where no action needs to be taken (Jones, 2021). This standard is so well established in the material world that surrounds us that, even without knowing about the standard itself, we instantly recognize these meanings. The change from red to green therefore has a direct impact on how effective the two messages are likely to be at dis/encouraging particular behaviours. This is reflected in comments on LinkedIn about whether the message in Figure 4.2 is encouraging direct action or not.

The fields of Multimodality and Social Semiotics (often used as analytical tools in CDA) deal with meanings that arise from combinations of communicative modes – be they verbal, visual, kinetic, aural – in particular cultural contexts. A multimodal approach to language and communication argues that we can only understand communication fully if we pay attention to all the modes involved, how these interact, and how they tend to get used more generally in different contexts. The latter idea captures the notion of connotative or associative meaning: that meanings arise not just from what semiotic signs refer to, but also carry social, affective, and evaluative components from the contexts in which we often encounter them. Because public health messages typically consist of highly multimodal texts (e.g. print posters, social media posts, radio or TV ads, etc.), Multimodal analysis is another useful framework for making sense of how they communicate their meanings. We discuss studies using multimodal analysis in sections 4.3.1 and 4.3.3.

4.1.1 Defining public health communication

Charles Edward Winslow, a theoretician and leader of public health in the United States in the 1920s, defined it as:

> the science and the art of preventing disease, prolonging life, and promoting physical health and efficiency through organised community efforts for the sanitation of the environment, the control of community infections, the education of the individual in principles of personal hygiene, the organisation of medical and nursing services for the early diagnosis and preventative treatment of disease, and the development of the social machinery which will ensure to every individual in the community a standard of living adequate for the maintenance of health.
>
> *(Winslow, 1920)*

You can see from this definition just how many potential stakeholders – with potentially competing interests – are involved in the area of public health. In this chapter we are most interested in how public health institutions inform, educate, empower, and encourage the public to change behaviours.

The ways in which these mainly communicative functions are performed differs widely around the world. Communications can include everything from the easily recognizable genre of a government or health authority sponsored print or radio 'public service announcement' (PSA) (such as those discussed in sections 4.3.1 and 4.3.3), to the much more implicit entertainment-education (EE) campaigns where public health messages are embedded in the plot of popular entertainment shows for different audiences. In between these two poles are individualized text messages, newspaper and magazine articles on health (as in section 4.3.2), illness and health-related websites and forums, patient information leaflets, user-generated health content, such as a tweet by a celebrity encouraging people to wear masks, and many more. Among the many challenges of public health communication is reaching the community that you intend to reach, and addressing them in a way that is effective for them (Neuhauser & Kreps, 2010, Tang & Rundblad, 2021).

4.1.2 In this chapter

Here we focus on types of public health communication that are widely used and easily accessible to those new to the field. We look at public health campaigns originating from national governments (sections 4.3.1 and 4.3.3), and public health communication in the form of newspaper articles (section 4.3.2). The media (including social media) are important vehicles and catalysts for public discourses of health, providing a link between official authorities and some sections of the wider public.

4.2 Preliminary considerations

In this section, we start with the decisions you have to make and issues you have to consider if you intend to conduct a study of language and communication in the context of public health. This complements the more general advice in Chapters 2 and 3.

4.2.1 Deciding the focus of your analysis

Public health communication data brings with it lots of very interesting questions that you can explore through linguistic analysis. Many students, when they first look at a piece of public health communication, will immediately want to assess whether it is effective or not. But the question of effectiveness is actually quite complicated, as discussed above: what exactly does that mean? There are lots of different ways that effectiveness can be operationalized (see Glik, 2007 for an overview) and some of these are amenable to linguistic analysis (e.g. whether a message is clear, involves creativity and is attention-grabbing), but others are not (e.g. whether a message is effective at creating behaviour change). Discourse analysis or multimodal analysis, where you look at how the text is itself constructed can help you describe what the language is like and *how* it communicates. You can then make predictions, or form hypotheses on the basis of what you know about how language works. For example, El Refaie argues that metaphors can be effective in public health messages, but different metaphors have to cohere with each other and with people's experiences more broadly, as you will see in section 4.3.3. You can also ask people directly, for example in surveys, interviews, or focus groups where you give people particular examples of public health communication data and capture their responses (e.g. McClaughlin et al. (2022) mentioned below, and the reader response studies mentioned in Chapter 5).

Other questions you might ask in relation to public health communication, which are answerable via linguistic methods, include what kinds of participants are represented in a message and what are they (supposed to be) doing? You could also ask questions about how a particular disease or public health issue is 'framed' or represented by messages. Is the disease presented as having autonomy and agency? What does that imply for how we need to approach it? For example, Collins et al. (2018) below argue that people's sense of individual responsibility for reducing antimicrobial resistance is understandably low, since media communications seem to diffuse responsibility to the societal level. You might then also ask *why* participants or diseases are represented in the way that they are. Mulderrig (2017) below, for example, talks about the alignment between presenting individuals as responsible for their own health and neoliberal ideologies.

4.2.2 Selecting public health communication data

One of the most common questions that students ask when they embark on their own research is 'how much data should I be collecting and analyzing?' As frustrating as that is, there really is no simple answer because many different factors impact how much data you can or should collect (see Chapter 2 for an overview). So perhaps a better place to start is asking not *how much*, but *what kind of* data to collect. The first thing you need to do is come up with different ways that you could categorize data that might be relevant to your questions.

The most obvious category, and one which we also discuss in Chapter 2, is the specific disease or public health issue, e.g. HIV/AIDS, obesity, breastfeeding, or indeed, Covid-19. The next category you might want to consider is to do with text type or genre. You could decide to focus only on print media such as billboards, posts on a social media platform, or embedded story lines in EE campaigns. You could also categorize your data options in terms of who is producing the text or who the intended audience is. You might want to focus only on public health messages issued by a government and aimed at women, for example. In most cases, in order to be systematic about what data you actually end up focusing on, you will need to combine several of these categories. If you're doing a comparative study, then you'll also need to decide which of these category variables you 'manipulate', and which ones you keep constant. For example, Brookes et al.'s (2016) study below focuses on breast- and bottle-feeding advice (two related health issues for comparison) for new mothers (same target audience) in the UK (same location), issued by the UK Department of Health (same originator) in the form of two leaflets (same genre).

4.3 Selected studies

The rest of this chapter will summarize concrete examples of linguistic analyses of different types of public health communication texts. The studies we review mostly follow the traditions of Multimodal Discourse Analysis, Critical Discourse Analysis, and a combination of the two, with different aspects of language and phenomena being the focus.

4.3.1 Agency and responsibility in public health campaigns

In this section we discuss two studies that question and explore the motivations behind and implications of public health campaigns for different groups of people, motivated by the theoretical framework of CDA and operationalizing their analyses in different ways. We begin with Brookes et al. (2016), who explore a UK public health campaign focused on infant feeding.

Take a look at the front covers of two feeding guides (information leaflets) briefly mentioned in Chapter 1.

The Off to the Best Start (Figure 4.4) leaflet consists of 23 pages and outlines the health benefits of breastfeeding, providing advice on how to do it and how to recognize signs that a baby is feeding well. The Guide to Bottle Feeding pamphlet (Figure 4.5) is a 21-page document with information and advice specifically on formula feeding. The documents were produced by the UK's Department of Health and UNICEF's Baby Friendly Initiative to help parents-to-be and families with babies and young children adopt healthy behaviours and build parenting skills (Public Health England).

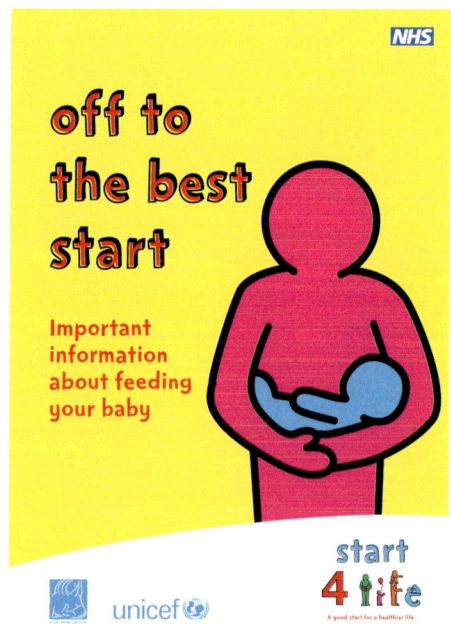

FIGURE 4.4   Breastfeeding Leaflet

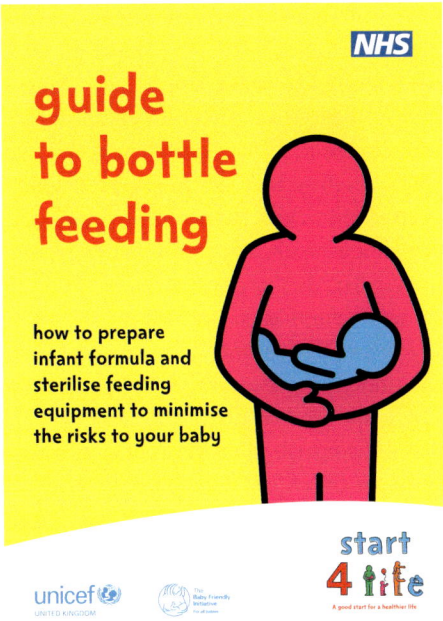

FIGURE 4.5   Formula feeding leaflet

Brookes et al. (2016) use critical multimodal discourse analysis (CMDA) to identify, among other things, how mothers are represented verbally and visually across the two texts. For example, they find that, in Off to the Best Start, mothers are often referred to as 'mum', while this reference is entirely absent from A Guide to Bottle Feeding. Instead, the latter uses the second-person pronoun 'you' and one instance of 'mother'. The authors argue that while 'mother' tends to index a biological role, 'mum' indexes a social role, so its use serves to strengthen the connection between what it means to be a mother at the societal level and breastfeeding. This more social and personalized view is supported by the different visuals chosen across the two texts. In A Guide to Bottle Feeding mothers tend to be depicted in depersonalizing ways, e.g. in photographs showing only the hands performing the tasks associated with preparing infant formula. When the mother's face is in shot, she is not smiling and her gaze is not directed at the viewer, so there is little engagement suggested/invited with the audience. In Off to the Best Start on the other hand, mothers are often depicted in close-up photographs, from a frontal angle and at eye level, which signal a shared space and intimacy between them and the reader/viewer (cf. Kress & van Leeuwen, 2006).

Breastfeeding itself is represented differently from bottle feeding. The former is often mentioned in superlative terms (e.g. 'the *best* start for your baby'; '*perfect* and uniquely made for your growing baby's needs'; 'the *healthiest* way to feed your baby', our emphases), while infant formula is often described according to qualities it does not possess and/or things that have been done to it to make it better (e.g. 'made from cow's milk that has been treated to make it suitable'; 'doesn't contain the ingredients that help protect your baby from infection and disease'). These choices (and others that the authors discuss in more detail) across the two texts clearly present breastfeeding and breastfeeding mothers in a more favourable light. The authors argue that this strategy, while supported by scientific evidence for the benefits of breastfeeding, aligns with neoliberal values around motherhood. Neoliberalism refers to a particular ideology and is a concept often invoked in CDA studies. Neoliberal societies emphasize the role of the individual, in this case the mother, in taking responsibility for their own and their families' lives, including their health. The underlying assumption is that mothers can simply make the 'responsible' or 'right' choice to breastfeed and thereby avert health risks. One problem with this is that it disregards the myriad of factors that might impact a mother's decision or ability to breastfeed, such as pain or other difficulties breastfeeding, the short duration of maternity leave, pressure from others not to breastfeed, and so on. Many of these factors are social, economic, or otherwise outside the individual mother's control. Therefore, the authors argue, presenting breastfeeding as a matter of personal choice puts an unfair amount of responsibility on mothers, potentially leading to the stigmatization of those who choose to or have to bottle-feed.

A similar approach to analysis, though with emphasis on verbal language, was taken by Mulderrig (2017) in relation to an anti-obesity public health campaign. Mulderrig examined the launch advert of 'Change4Life' – a long-term social marketing campaign to support a governmental strategy tackling childhood obesity in England (cf. DoH, 2008). She compared it with UK governmental policy documents and underpinning social practices to ascertain how it uses language to encourage compliance with desired policies, while retaining (a sense of) freedom of choice.

The example below, is the transcript of the TV advert that launched the campaign on UK television in 2009:

EXAMPLE 4.1

1. Once upon a time life was pretty simple. It could be hard: the food was pretty fast, but it could
2. be fun, if we got our mammoth or bison, or whatever.
3. *[Cheers as a monster is clubbed].*
4. *[Images moving towards an urbanised environment and a 'window' into modern family life*
5. *eating fast food and snacking in front of the TV]*
6. Then, gradually life changed. In many ways it got easier: nobody had to run around for their food.

7.   Or anything else much for that matter.

8.   *[Images of child's 'insides' and fat build-up]*

9.   Until one day we woke up and realised that 9 out of 10 of our kids would grow up to have

10.   dangerous amounts of fat build up in their bodies, which meant they're more likely to get

11.   horrid things like heart disease, diabetes, and cancer.

12.   *[Computer game on-screen exterminates figure of child. Parent and child exclaim in horror]*

13.   And many can have their lives cut short.

14.   *[Cut to the picnic in the park scene. Figures adopt acrobatic poses to form the words 'eat',*

15.   *'move' and 'live', then run into the final scene to form part of the brand logo]*

16.   So we thought that's not MORE of a life, that's LESS of a life, and that's TERRIBLE, cos

17.   we love the little blighters

18.   Maybe we should get together with our kids and eat better, move more, live longer, and

19.   change for life

20.   And we all lived happily, not exactly ever after, but more ever after, than we had done.

21.   To find out how you can change for life, search online for Change4Life.

(The video of the ad can be found at www.youtube.com/watch?v=yJAnnHJRGsI)

The historical narrative (with intertextual references to fairytales like 'Once upon a time') spoken by a male voice-over locates the source of the problem of obesity in modern consumer lifestyles. Focusing in on lines 9–13, Mulderrig examines how the health-related facts are reported in the advert in contrast to the policy documents and reports that informed it (namely, the Foresight Report, Butland et al., 2007, and 'Healthy Weight, Healthy Lives', DoH, 2008). Table 4.1 below provides an overview of what health facts are contained in the reports and, in the final row, how they've been reproduced in the TV ad.

Mulderrig (2017) notes three transformations in the way that key biomedical information is reported from official reports to the TV ad: exaggerated statistics, simplified and emotive biomedical facts, and vague health categories.

The TV ad makes the shocking statistical claim that 9 out 10 children will be affected by obesity in the future. This is a much larger percentage than is claimed by either of the governmental reports, which talk about '25%' and almost 'two-thirds' of children. The extreme formulation in the advert is possible because neither the age range involved, nor the meaning of 'dangerous levels of fat' are specified. Even in the Change4Life policy document itself, the '9 out of 10' statistic is expressed as 'only one in ten' adults predicted to be a 'healthy weight'. The 'flipping' of the statistic to be about children is problematic because causal links between childhood weight and adult weight are difficult to establish. But the focus on children in the ad does make the future much more alarming.

Similarly, while the Foresight report focused on the category of obesity (which is biomedically defined as a body-mass-index (BMI) of 30 to 39.9), the TV ad simply talks about 'dangerous levels of fat in the body'. This is because market research in the commissioning of the advert revealed that official BMI categories like 'obese' and 'overweight' were off-putting for people. Sacrificing accuracy here, enabled the exaggerated statistical claims outlined above. A further distortion in the TV ad is that biomedical risks are reported in a simplified way, with fewer diseases cited, and using more informal register (e.g. 'kids', 'horrid things', 'one day we woke up and realized'), and emotive language (e.g. 'severe impact', 'life-threatening'). These types of language are particularly persuasive because they tap into people's private anxieties and aim to use those to achieve behaviour change.

This kind of side-by-side comparative analysis is an effective way to evidence claims about inaccuracies and misleading representations in linguistic research. It ensures that you, as a language researcher, go beyond simply claiming that scientific and health-related information is distorted and over-simplified (cf. Jones, 2013) and instead enables you to show *how* it is so.

Mulderrig also examines how different social actors are represented in the TV ad. She starts by outlining how the Foresight report in particular, which supposedly underpins the Change4Life policy and campaign, goes to some lengths to outline the various societal and economic factors implicated in rising levels of

TABLE 4.1 Adapted from Mulderrig 2017: 'Table 1. Recontextualization of biomedical facts about obesity across policy texts'

Report/Source	Content/Fact
Foresight report, 2007	By 2050 approximately 25% of under-20-year-olds are predicted to be obese. (36) Being overweight or obese increases the risk of a wide range of chronic diseases, principally type 2 diabetes, hypertension, cardiovascular disease including stroke, as well as cancer.
Foresight 'Summary of Key Messages', 2007	By 2050 [...] about 25% of all children under 16 could be obese. (2) Obesity increases the risk of a range of chronic diseases, particularly type 2 diabetes, stroke and coronary heart disease and also cancer and arthritis.
Healthy Weight, Healthy Lives, 2008	[the numbers of people either overweight or obese] could rise to almost nine in ten adults and two-thirds of children by 2050. (pvii) This trend [obesity] increases has a severe impact on the health of individuals increasing the risk of diabetes, cancer and heart and liver disease.
Change4Life Launch advert, January 2009	One day we woke up and realized that 9 out of 10 of our kids would grow up to have dangerous amounts of fat build up in their bodies, which meant they're more likely to get horrid things like heart disease, diabetes, and cancer.

obesity. The TV ad begins with a hint of this when it focuses on modern life-styles as underlying the problem. In this section, social actors are represented by an inclusive 'we', i.e. the pronoun obviously includes both the speaker and the addressee. However, at the point where scientific facts are about to be relayed (line 9), the plural first-person pronouns become more ambiguous. In line 9, 'we' must refer only to the government since they are the ones who commission and read the reports on which the following information is based. However, the pronoun in 'our kids' refers to the general public as well as the government. The same kind of slippage occurs in lines 16–17 where the negative view of the future is evaluated by the exclusive 'we' that does not include the audience ('we thought that's not more of a life' …), followed by an inclusive 'we' ('cos we love the little blighters'). Finally, the actions to be taken to avoid the negative future are all to be done by an inclusive 'we', but the actions themselves have to be performed at the individual not the societal level. This is made explicit in the final line with a switch to 'you'.

Mulderrig argues that such linguistic strategies recontextualize and simplify the issue of obesity, in a way that makes it seem like an individual problem requiring individualized solutions. The problem, as with breastfeeding, is that obesity is in fact highly complex and interlinked with a number of social, economic, and otherwise structural issues (e.g. poverty). Mulderrig therefore sees the particular techniques employed by the Change4Life campaign as very much part of the same neoliberal agenda that Brookes et al. (2016) noted above, which ultimately defines a social problem in individualized terms and thereby limits governmental, while increasing personal responsibility for addressing it.

The types of public health campaigns outlined in this section are examples of social marketing, where techniques from the private sector, specifically advertising and marketing, are used to achieve public sector goals (e.g. governmental or public health policy). Critical analyses, whether of verbal (CDA) or multimodal content (CMDA), are particularly appropriate for examining these complex interrelations because their very aim is to uncover the assumptions, motivations, and power structures that underpin and are perpetuated by these communications. At the same time, you do have to be cautious when discussing intentions or motivations behind public health messages. With the specific methodologies outlined in the studies above, it is simply not possible to make clear-cut or categorical claims about these. You can hypothesize on the basis of patterns and wider contextual information and ideologies, like Mulderrig and Brookes et al. above. But it is important to be aware of the limitations of the methods you are using: textual linguistic analysis does not tell you directly about what assumption and intentions motivated a particular health message.

You also need to bear in mind how complex the domain of public health is, and therefore the many different objectives, audiences, stakeholders, time pressures that need to be balanced in different communications, involving potentially multiple authors. In these circumstances even messages that are generally beneficial to the public, or overall well-meaning, can end up stigmatizing some groups or ignoring the conditions that affect the way they live their lives.

Of course, it is also perfectly acceptable to conduct analyses on public health campaigns that are not aimed at uncovering assumptions, motivations, and power structures, but rather at simply identifying patterns of representation. Thompson (2012), for example, conducted a multimodal analysis of how people with mental illness are represented on a website, using Kress and van Leeuwen's (1996) social semiotic framework. Others have looked at the use (or lack) of minority languages in public health communications (e.g. Piller et al., 2020), since such texts should – in theory – speak to all groups in a population. You can also investigate how such (lack of) representation might relate to people's attitudes and behaviours. It is to these kinds of studies, specifically in news media, that we turn in the next section.

4.3.2 Risk and uncertainty in media reporting

Around the world, news media have been shown to impact public understanding of health issues (e.g. Trumbo, 2012). Unsurprisingly, as the main link between health, governmental and other institutional authorities and the general publics, the media have a large role to play in guiding perceptions, attitudes and behaviour. Among the main aspects of health issues that the media often report on are the degrees of risk and uncertainty around health threats, diseases, and health interventions. But communicating about risks is difficult because, even when risk can be specified, as a percentage for example, the significance of that risk for any particular individual (and therefore how likely they are to change their behaviour to mitigate it) will vary according to cognitive, emotional, interpersonal, contextual, and societal factors (Waters et al., 2014). Any uncertainty around risks further exacerbates this problem because it also affects 'how people perceive a risk, how they interpret information about it, how motivated they will be to take actions in response to it, and how much they trust the people and institutions responsible for managing it' (Paek & Hove, 2020: 1730).

Tang and Rundbland (2020) investigated precisely this role of uncertainty in the reporting of the health risks of endocrine-disrupting compounds (EDCs) and pharmaceuticals and personal care products (PPCPs) found in drinking water. To illustrate the different ways in which uncertainty can manifest and the consequences this can have for people's perception of risk, the authors compared how press releases by the water industry and regulatory bodies 'entextualize' risks with how these are 'recontextualized' in media reports (cf. Briggs & Baumann, 1990). Using terminology from Cognitive Linguistics (e.g. Ungerer & Schmid, 2006), Tang and Rundblad (2020) demonstrated how different participants are portrayed in the two types of texts. In this way, they showed how small risks to health reported by water industry and regulatory experts can end up being perceived as potentially large risks by the public. A key factor is un/certainty communicated via im/precision in language.

Compare the level of precision with which water contaminants and their effects are represented in the two examples below from Tang and Rundblad (2020):

EXAMPLE 4.2

What are 'PPCPs'?

These are pharmaceuticals and personal care products used for personal health or cosmetic reasons or used by agricultural businesses to enhance growth or health of livestock. PPCPs include thousands of prescription and over-the-counter therapeutic drugs, veterinary drugs, fragrances, lotions and cosmetics. People contribute PPCPs to the environment when medication passes out of the body and into sewer lines, external products wash down the bath drain or when unused medication is placed in the trash.

Is my water safe?

Studies have shown that pharmaceuticals are present at extremely low levels in our water supplies. Further research suggests that certain drugs may cause ecological harm. More research is needed to determine if PPCPs have potential human health effects. To date, scientists have found no evidence of adverse human health effects from PPCPs in the environment. (Virginia Department of Health)

EXAMPLE 4.3

In tests of wastewater retrieved near other European hospitals and one in Davis County, Utah, scientists were able to link drug dumping to virulent antibiotic-resistant germs and genetic mutations that may promote cancers, according to scientific studies reviewed by the AP.

Researchers have focused on cell-poisoning anticancer drugs and fluoroquinolone class antibiotics, like anthrax fighter ciprofloxacin.

At the University of Rouen Medical Center in France, 31 of 38 wastewater samples showed the ability to mutate genes. A Swiss study of hospital wastewater suggested that fluoroquinolone antibiotics also can disfigure bacterial DNA, raising the question of whether such drug concoctions can heighten the risk of cancer in humans.

(Associated Press, April 2008)

Example 4.2 comes from a government department responsible for public health policy and involved in regulating the water industry, while Example 4.3 is a news media article produced by Associated Press.

Tang and Rundblad (2020) show that, in water industry and regulatory texts, like Example 4.2, contaminants are often referred to in semantically precise ways (e.g. 'PPCP') and sometimes further specified via listing (e.g. 'veterinary drugs, fragrances, lotions and cosmetics'). The consequences themselves, however, tend to be reported in less semantically precise ways (e.g. 'may cause *ecological harm*'; 'if

PPCPs have potential *human health effects*', emphasis in the original). Although it is implied that wildlife and humans are potentially at risk, the exact nature of the threat, the effect, remains vague (e.g. 'harm', 'effect'). The authors explain this pattern by the fact that, at the time of writing, the existence of contaminants in the water supply was uncontested and quantifiable, but the exact nature of their effects and who or what might be at risk was uncertain.

In media texts (like Example 4.3), the reporting of the effects of contaminants was somewhat different. Across different media texts, the possible health effects of these water contaminants were reported in more specific terms. This can be seen in the contrast between 'risk of cancer' in Example 4.3 and 'potential human health effects' in the industry text, while further specific references in other media texts included 'virulent antibiotic-resistant germs' and 'genetic mutations'. In these and other patterns, the authors found an overriding tendency for a heightened specificity when it comes to expressing the potential harmfulness of contaminants in media texts. Specificity implies certainty. At the same time, references to the contaminants themselves were less semantically precise. These tended to be referred to with vaguer, more everyday terms such as drugs', 'chemicals' and 'compounds'. Although the scientific uncertainty about the likelihood of harm was communicated in some ways (mostly through modal verbs of uncertainty, like 'can'), the authors argue that the combination with more specific health harms underplayed the level of scientific uncertainty and possibly contributed to inconsistency within the media articles themselves. This left room for a wider range of interpretations.

In effect, media texts inverted the certainty patterns of industry texts: while the latter communicated certainty about what contaminants were but less certainty about their effects; the former communicated certainty about effects, but less precision in what the contaminants were. This is another good example of public health communication research that relies on comparisons between different types of texts focused on the same issue. Since linguistic representation involves making a choice between different sets of viable options, each option 'acquires its meanings against the background of other choices which could have been made' (Eggins, 2004: 3). Comparing two choices that were made can help us understand the implications of one versus another. Tang and Rundblad (2020) examine a range of other linguistic characteristics in water industry and media texts, but one of their key concerns is that the more room there is for audiences to infer information, connections and likelihoods, the greater the chance of miscommunication. In this case, the public seemed to over-estimate the relevance and risks to themselves. In the following study media portrayals of different participants in the context of antimicrobial resistance, seem to have the opposite effect.

Using the tools of Systemic Functional Linguistics (SFL) (e.g. Thompson, 2013), rather than Cognitive Linguistics, Collins et al. (2018) focus on communications in the UK news media. As we briefly mentioned in Chapter 1, they are concerned with the health threat of antimicrobial resistance (AMR), which refers to a global concern that microbes (e.g. bacteria, fungi, etc.) are increasingly evolving mechanisms that protect them from the effects of antimicrobials, such as antibiotics. The causes of AMR are multifaceted and complex, but include, along with agricultural and pharmacological practices, people's individual use and overuse of antibiotics. Yet, there appears to be an assumption among the general public that AMR is an issue that 'ordinary people' have no control over (cf. McCulloch et al., 2016), which can mean that people are less motivated to change behaviours to prevent or reduce AMR.

Collins et al. were interested in finding out whether this assumption could be linked to media communications about AMR, especially with regard to clarity about who should be taking what kind of action. They explored which social actors, or participants, are represented as having agency around antimicrobial resistance, and what kind of agency they have, i.e. what are they represented as doing. Consider Example 4.4 below:

EXAMPLE 4.4

> Antibiotics are used on farms, on livestock, under the prescription and care of a veterinary surgeon.
>
> (*The Independent, 20 June 2011*, cited in
> Collins et al., 2018)

In the SFL approach that the authors apply, the focus is on who or what (participant) is represented as doing what (process) to whom (participant), when, where and how (circumstances associated with the process). This is known as the 'ideational metafunction' of language in Systemic Functional Linguistics, i.e. the systems in language that represent the world around us. SFL focuses on the functional role that different components of a clause perform in a sentence, regardless of their syntactic position. The idea, introduced earlier, that linguistic representation is a choice between different options for making meaning is actually based on a claim by M.A.K Halliday, who is one of the founding scholars of SFL (Halliday, 1972). In the example above, the process is 'used' and the thing being used is 'antibiotics' (i.e. it is the participant that is affected by the process). It is not explicit who does the using due to the passive structure (although we can guess that it's farmers). Because 'antibiotics' is in the subject position of the sentence, but it is not the participant doing the action, we can say that the active or 'agentive' participants are backgrounded or hidden. The same event could, however, also be represented as follows: 'Farmers use antibiotics on farms on livestock, when a veterinary surgeon prescribes them'. If the author of the *Independent* article had chosen this linguistic representation, then both farmers and veterinary surgeons would be more explicitly presented as agentive participants, i.e. the ones responsible for the use of antibiotics.

Agency, as applied in Collins et al., refers first to the 'grammatical agency' of participants, i.e. their syntactic role in a sentence. Participants in subject position, in this definition, have agency, while participants in object position do not. In addition, Collins et al. also consider 'semantic agency', which refers to the extent to which participants are represented as effecting change. This kind of agency is a matter of degree, and can be deduced from the types of processes that participants are involved in.

Collins et al. (2018) focused on 627 articles from 16 national newspapers that included the words 'antibiotic resistance' or 'antimicrobial resistance' or 'superbug' between 2010 and 2015. With such a large quantity of data, the authors of course restricted their analysis to a very specific aspect of language, namely the participants and processes around any mentions of 'antibiotics'. They used corpus analysis software (for more on corpus analysis, see Chapters 2 and 7) to find all examples of the word 'antibiotics' in the dataset and then conducted a manual analysis for participants and processes that occurred around this 'node word'.

The main types of participants, or social actors, in subject position that the authors identified in this way can be labelled broadly as bacteria and infections, doctors and prescribers, patients and the general public, and the antibiotics themselves. The general public, the authors explain, is often referred to by the ambiguous first-person plural pronoun 'we' (as discussed in the context of Mulderrig, 2017 above). 'We' is used frequently across the texts and indicates a focus on the readers' agency and responsibility in the rise of AMR, potentially also suggesting that 'we' are to blame. This is not just because 'we' appears in subject position frequently (grammatical agency), but also because of the types of processes or activities that 'we' do (semantic agency). 'We' are the ones who 'demand' antibiotics from our doctors, who 'use', and should 'reduce' our use of them. In SFL, 'use' and 'reduce' are categorized as 'material' processes because they effect a change in the environment or create something that wasn't there before. For this reason, they denote high semantic agency. 'Demand' denotes a moderate degree of agency (in SFL, it is called a 'verbal' process), because someone is usually affected by the activity, i.e. someone hears or reads what we demand, but it doesn't effect change as directly as material processes. However, Collins et al. note that, while 'we' are presented as responsible for AMR to some extent, the ambiguity in the plural pronoun 'we' means that there are no real implications for individual responsibility. As a reference to social actors, 'we' is just too broad. This presents AMR as a general societal issue that individual people or groups have no control over.

Furthermore, AMR is also presented as a biological problem when high levels of agency are attributed to the infections that antibiotics fight. These 'bacteria' and 'superbugs' are presented as 'developing' into forms that 'survive' and 'evade' antibiotic treatment, almost as if they had free will. Because agency tends to entail responsibility, this also suggests that the bacteria themselves are to blame for AMR, thereby reducing any sense of personal responsibility that individuals might feel even further.

As with many other health and science topics, mainstream media has a great deal of influence on the general public's awareness and perceptions of this issue. If the public are referred to in ambiguous or very broad terms, especially when faced with social actors who are referred to more specifically and given more semantic agency, then it is no wonder that the public perceive themselves as without individual responsibility for reducing the potential for AMR to develop. Such public perceptions can play a fundamental role in how people behave in relation to antibiotics and other health threats. As noted both at the beginning of this section and in the introduction, clarity and precision (about the right things) in public health communication are paramount. And it is not only the traditional media that can have this kind of influence. Social media platforms such as Twitter, Weibo, Facebook, and TikTok (at the time of writing) increasingly serve as sources of information on health-related topics. Similar analyses, looking at the representation of conditions or health issues, can therefore be conducted on data gathered from these channels as well. In addition, these sources of data can also be used to explore public reactions to official representations and get a sense of user-generated concerns relating to specific topics.

4.3.3 *The* potential *effectiveness of public health campaigns*

In this final section we want to address that complicated issue of 'effectiveness' in public health communication we flagged at the beginning of this chapter. It is our experience that students often wish to establish whether a public health message or campaign is effective or not, even though linguistic methods are often unsuitable for this purpose. With this in mind, we want to suggest how something along these lines can be done; how *potential* effectiveness can be approached or approximated through linguistic analysis. While not necessarily assessing whether people in fact attend and respond to a public health message as intended, linguistic analysis can be used to explore how a particular message is designed and whether this design appears coherent, attention-grabbing, and appropriate to a given audience and context. The underlying assumption is that if these design principles are in place, then a message is *more likely to be* effective. In this section we return to communicative resources in multiple modes (especially verbal and visual) and how they can be deployed in public health communication.

Consider the poster in Figure 4.6.

Oyebode and Unuabonah (2013) describe how the visual and verbal resources combine in this poster to make it appropriate for the target audience and the intended message. Drawing on Kress and van Leeuwen's (1996) visual grammar, the authors note that the central image depicts a happy, traditional Yoruba family, with a smiling mother, father, and two children. The Yoruba live in southwestern Nigeria where this poster was displayed in the waiting area of an HIV/AIDS clinic of a state hospital. More specifically, the dress code of the family depicted signals that they are a rural, lower-class family.

The combination of this image with the theme or primary announcement 'HIV Prevention for People Living with HIV/AIDS' connotes a sense of hope that people living with HIV/AIDS can raise happy families, even if they hail

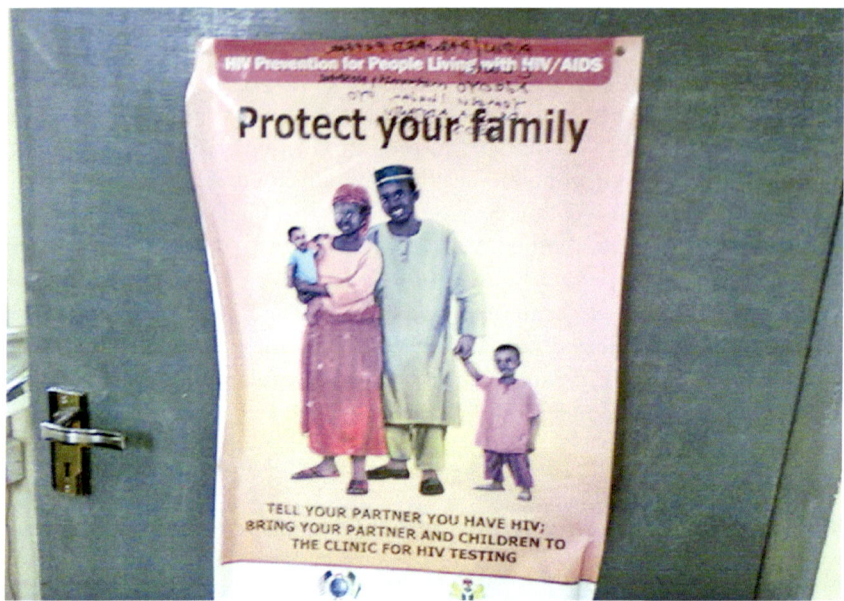

FIGURE 4.6 HIV prevention poster from Nigeria

from rural or lower-class backgrounds. The means to achieve this is outlined in the secondary announcements to 'Protect your family' by telling them about your HIV status and getting them tested. These verbal instructions are once again supported by the visual grammar of the image. Oyebode and Unuabonah (2013) argue that the frontal angle and direct gaze of the people depicted invites involvement and engagement. Similarly to the verbal text (especially with 'you' and 'your'), it directly addresses the audience and signals that they should take action.

The frame of the image is that of a 'long shot' from which point of view the whole person can be seen. This signals a certain distance that can be suggestive of objectivity or factuality. The authors argue that this indicates the truth value of the message, whether audiences choose to believe it or not. A sense of authority is also conveyed by the use of imperatives and the Nigerian coat of arms, which positions the sender of the message as institutionally powerful. However, Oyebode and Unuabonah (2013) suggest that the eye-level angle of the image helps to offset this imbalance slightly by signalling more equality between addresser and addressee.

The authors suggest that in the specific local context in which this poster (and others like it) appeared, this combination of visual and verbal resources manages to strike a balance between authoritativeness and approachability, communicating hope and the need to take action. It manages to counter negative perceptions of people living with HIV/AIDS while also emphasizing the need to take precautions. These features mean that the text has been designed to achieve the particular effects outlined and it is therefore *potentially* effective at doing so. But actual effectiveness is not, and cannot be, measured by this textual analysis alone.

A different approach to message effectiveness in public health campaigns is taken by El Refaie (2015). She focuses on the phenomenon of metaphor (both verbal and multimodal) and starts by summarizing what we know about the effects of metaphor as a communicative tool. What is its role in persuasion, for example? She quotes a meta-analysis by Sopory and Dillard (2002) which concluded that there is evidence of a persuasive effect of metaphor (i.e. it can be effective at persuading), but only if certain conditions are met, such as audience familiarity with the topic (what a metaphor is trying to describe), the metaphor being novel or creative, but also simple. El Refaie argues that metaphors in public health campaigns involving new or complex information additionally have to have coherence. They have to cohere with each other (where different metaphors are used), and crucially, with people's cultural understandings and experiences.[1] Coherence in this sense has been shown to reduce the risk of misunderstandings. So here the question of whether a text is effective or not actually becomes: are these conditions of coherence met in a particular instance of public health communication? In other words, one way of approaching questions of effectiveness is to use the findings of experimental research to assess the impact of the linguistic features of a specific text.

Let's look at one of the examples discussed by El Refaie (2015), *Laduma* (Figure 4.7). *Laduma* is an A4 booklet consisting of eight full-colour pages of a comic strip and activities around prevention and treatment of tuberculosis (TB) aimed at children. It was initiated by the Centers for Disease Control and Prevention, Global AIDS Program, South Africa, and the Eastern Cape Department of Health with funding from the US President's Emergency Plan for AIDS Relief and produced by the South African Jive Media. Copies were distributed through public health facilities, charities, and national and provincial departments of health in South Africa.

Set in a small village in South Africa, the comic strip tells the story of Themba, a young boy, who suddenly performs badly in a soccer match despite being the best scorer of the team. His teammate, Thandi, asks him what's wrong and he describes not feeling well and coughing. Thandi recognizes these as symptoms of TB and persuades Themba to go to the clinic for antibiotics and for advice on how to regain his health and avoid passing the illness on to others. Themba follows the guidance, and scores the winning goal for his team at a match a few weeks later (Figure 4.8). The activities in the booklet reinforce some of the advice that Themba receives in the story: there is a maze that leads to a clinic, a crossword puzzle which hides the symptoms of TB, and an activity that gets children to grow their own beans, which they can eat as part of the healthy diet that helps people recover more quickly.

El Refaie focuses on the overarching soccer metaphor, which is realized in verbal metaphors such as 'gameplan', and the parallel set up between winning at soccer and recovering from tuberculosis (TB) in the final statement by one of the

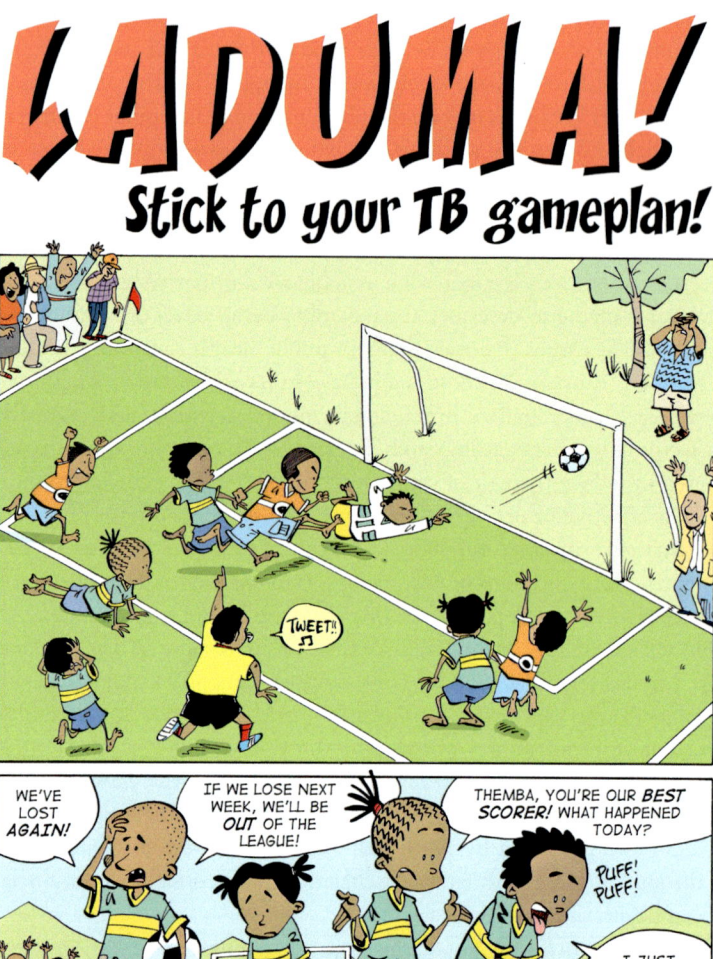

FIGURE 4.7 Laduma! Cover (Credit: Jive Media)

characters: 'You see – success is all about commitment. That is how you win on the soccer field and how you beat TB too!' The same metaphor is also realized multimodally in the literal soccer story being told.

El Refaie argues that this central soccer metaphor coheres with the audience's cultural experience because regular training is something that most children in South Africa have experience with. This concrete, physical experience is used to help children understand the more abstract concept of how to recover from TB. The metaphor is also internally coherent in that different aspects of soccer

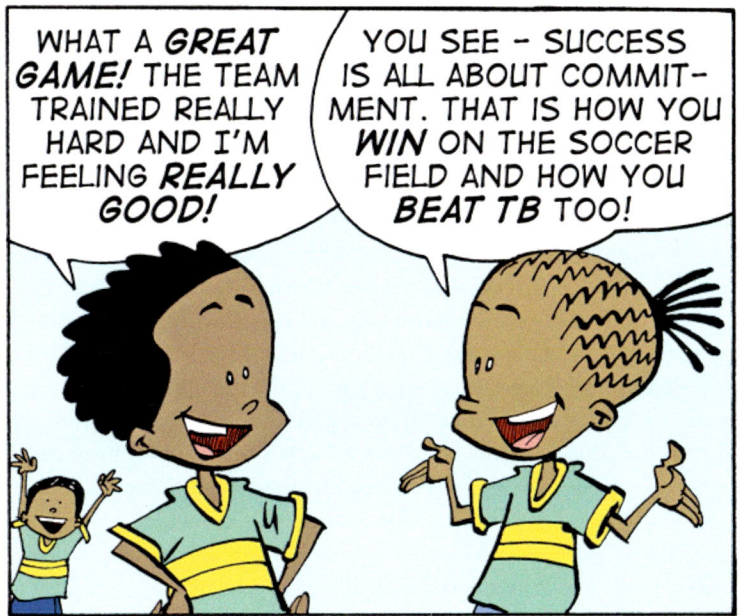

FIGURE 4.8   Laduma final panel (Credit: Jive Media)

training map neatly onto different aspects of TB recovery (e.g. suddenly playing badly and falling ill; the need for physical commitment and effort and mental commitment and effort to improve; playing together as a team and collectively preventing the spread of TB; playing well again and recovery). Some elements of this are also realized in the activities that children are encouraged to complete: for example, all activities are easy to complete and therefore are also a form of playing. And this playing involves doing things that will help children recover from TB.

But the booklet also involves metaphors other than soccer. For example, the plant growing metaphor is instantiated in the bean growing activity and made explicit in the simile 'Getting better from TB takes a long time – like plants which take time to grow but give us food in the end' towards the end of the booklet. This metaphor is again coherent with children's everyday experiences, and it coheres with the central soccer metaphor too. It draws on an activity that is pleasurable and playful, but highlights better a different aspect of the TB experience. The plant metaphor emphasizes the patience and persistence required in regularly taking medication. These characteristics also apply to soccer training, and are therefore consistent with it, but are perhaps less salient in the latter.

El Refaie's main point is that these types of metaphor coherence are essential in health campaigns that want to communicate new and often complex information. In this sense whether metaphors in a health campaign cohere or not can be seen as a factor in their potential effectiveness.

It is worth bearing in mind that, as we outlined in the introduction to the chapter, assessing the actual effectiveness of a public health campaign is complicated, depends on how one defines effectiveness, and usually requires methods other than, or in addition to, linguistic analysis. In this section, we have therefore outlined ways in which potential/hypothetical effectiveness can be approached or approximated. These types of analyses are important because they outline why certain ways of communicating *might* be effective in specific circumstances, but it is important to remember that they do not test whether they actually are effective or not when received by particular people and communities. Testing such hypotheses often involves experimental methods, as in Hendricks et al. (2018) where the researchers tested whether Journey and Battle metaphors describing a fictional experience of cancer lead to different appraisals of the fictional protagonist's situation. It can also be achieved in the context of large-scale projects by combining multiple methods of analysis – some discourse analytic, some not – as in McClaughlin et al. (2022). McClaughlin et al. (2022) combined corpus linguistic analysis (see Chapters 2 and 7) with a public survey and interactions with a Public Involvement Panel to explore how different types of Covid-19 related public health messages were received.

4.4 Concluding remarks

Public health communication is a group of genres that come in many different forms. These have to manage the potentially competing interests of multiple stakeholders and diverse audiences, which means that getting such communications 'right' can be very difficult. Public health communications and campaigns often bear traces of the tensions that underlie their production and as such can shed light on ideologies and hidden assumptions. They are also important to study because they have an impact of public perceptions and behaviour and behaviour around illness and disease.

Public health communications data can be easily accessible for students and early career researchers, making it particularly suitable for exploration in the context of dissertations and theses. However, it is important to bear in mind the wider cultural, temporal, but also discourse context of any 'texts' as these also play an important role in how they can be interpreted in the real world.

Note

1 El Refaie (2015) is careful to note that these are only appropriate conditions of persuasiveness in public health campaigns, partly because of their vast target audiences. They are not necessarily appropriate conditions or measures for other types of health communication, such as lived-experience accounts.

Further readings

Crichton, J., Candlin, C., & Firkins, A. S. (2016). *Communicating risk*. Palgrave Macmillan.

Jones, R. (Eds.). (2021). *Viral discourse: Doing discourse analysis in the midst of a pandemic*. Cambridge University Press.

Kress, G. R., & van Leeuwen, T. (2021). *Reading images: The grammar of visual design* (3rd ed.). Routledge.

References

Bauman, R., & Briggs, C. L. (1990). Poetics and performances as critical perspectives on language and social life. *Annual Review of Anthropology, 19*(1), 59–88.

Brookes, G., Harvey, K., & Mullany, L. (2016). 'Off to the best start'? A multimodal critique of breast and formula feeding health promotional discourse. *Gender and Language, 10*(3), 340–363.

Butland, B., Jebb, S., Kopelman, P., McPherson, K., Mardell, J., & Parry, V. (2007). *Foresight tackling obesities: Future choices – Project report* (2nd ed.). Government Office for Science. Retrieved May 27, 2016, from http://www.foresight.gov.uk/Obesity/17.pdf

Collins, L. C., Jaspal, R., & Nerlich, B. (2018). Who or what has agency in the discussion of antimicrobial resistance in UK news media (2010–2015)? A transitivity analysis. *Health, 22*(6), 521–540.

DH (Department of Health). (2008). *Healthy weight, healthy lives: A cross government strategy for England*. Central Office of Information.

Eggins, S. (2004). *An introduction to systemic functional linguistics* (2nd ed.). Continuum.

El Refaie, E. (2015). Scoring a goal or an own-goal against disease? A multilevel framework for describing metaphor coherence in health campaigns. *Metaphor and the Social World, 5*(1), 102–123.

Fairclough, N. (2001). *Language and power* (2nd ed.). Longman.

Fishbein, M., & Ajzen, I. (2010). *Predicting and changing behavior: The reasoned action approach*. Taylor & Francis.

Glik, D. C. (2007). Risk communication for public health emergencies. *Annual Review of Public Health, 28*(1), 33–54.

Halliday, M. A. K. (1972). Towards a sociological semantics. From the series of working papers and prepublications (14/C, 1972). Centre Internazionale di Semiotica e Linguistica of the University of Urbino

Hendricks, R. K., Demjén, Z., Semino, E., & Boroditsky, L. (2018). Emotional implications of metaphor: Consequences of metaphor framing for mindset about cancer. *Metaphor and Symbol, 33*(4), 267–279.

Jones, R. (2013). *Health and risk communication*. Routledge.

Jones, R. (2021). Order out of Chaos: Coronavirus communication and the construction of competence. In R. Jones (Ed.), *Viral discourse: Doing discourse analysis in the midst of a pandemic*. CUP.

Kress, G., & van Leeuwen, T. (1996). *Reading images: The grammar of visual design*. Routledge.

Kress, G., & van Leeuwen, T. (2006). *Reading images: The grammar of visual design*. (2nd ed.). Routledge.

McClaughlin, E., Vilar-Lluch, S., Parnell, T., Knight, D., Nichele, E., Adolphs, S. Clos, J., & Schiazza, G. (2022). The reception of public health messages during the COVID-19 pandemic. *Applied Corpus Linguistics* (Online First), *3*(1), 100037.

McCullough, A. R., Parekh, S., Rathbone, J., Del Mar, C. B, & Hoffmann, T. C. (2016). A systematic review of the public's knowledge and beliefs about antibiotic resistance. *Journal of Antimicrobial Chemotherapy*, *71*(1), 27–33.

Mulderrig, J. (2017). Reframing obesity: A critical discourse analysis of the UK's first social marketing campaign. *Critical Policy Studies*, *11*(4), 455–476.

Neuhauser, L., & Kreps, G. L. (2010). Ehealth communication and behavior change: Promise and performance. *Social Semiotics*, *20*(1), 9–27.

Oyebode, O., & Unuabonah, F. O. (2013). Coping with HIV/AIDS: A multimodal discourse analysis of selected HIV/AIDS posters in south-western Nigeria. *Discourse and Society*, *24*(6), 810–827.

Paek, H., & Hove, T. (2017). Risk perceptions and risk characteristics. *Oxford Research Encyclopedia of Communication*. Retrieved from https://oxfordre.com/communication /view/10.1093/acrefore/9780190228613.001.0001/acrefore-9780190228613-e-283

Piller, I., Zhang, J., & Li, J. (2020). Linguistic diversity in a time of crisis: Language challenges of the COVID-19 pandemic. *Multilingua*, *39*(5), 503–515.

Sopory, P., & Dillard, J. P. (2002). The persuasive effects of metaphor: A meta-analysis. *Human Communication Research*, *28*(3), 382–419.

Sridhar, D. (2022). *Preventable how a pandemic changed the world & how to stop the next one*. Penguin.

Tang, C., & Rundblad, G. (2020). A media brew of implied, hidden and unknown risk claims: Cognitive discourse analysis of public health communication. In Z. Demjén (Ed.), *Applying linguistics in illness and healthcare contexts*. Bloomsbury.

Tang, C., & Rundblad, G. (2021). *Mediation as a strategy for promoting COVID vaccination uptake amongst UK Bangladeshis (Project Report)*. Retrieved October 2022, from https://www.kcl.ac.uk/ecs/assets/projects/recommendations-for-promoting-vaccine -uptake-amongst-uk-bangladeshis.pdf

Thompson, G. (2013). *Introducing functional grammar* (3rd ed.). Routeldge.

Thompson, R. (2012). Looking healthy: Visualizing mental health and illness online. *Visual Communication*, *11*(4), 395–420.

Trumbo, C. W. (2012). The effect of newspaper coverage of influenza in the rate of physician visits for influenza 2002–2008. *Mass Communication and Society*, *15*(5), 718–738.

Ungerer, F., & Schmid, H.-J. (2006). *An introduction to cognitive linguistics* (2nd ed.). Routledge.

Waters, E. A., McQueen, A., & Cameron, L. D. (2014). Perceived risk and health risk communication. In H. Hamilton and W-Y. S. Chou (eds) *The Routledge handbook of language and health communication* London: Routledge.

Winslow, C. E. A. (1920). The untilled field of public health. *Modern Medicine*, *2*, 183–191.

Wright, L., Steptoe, A., & Fancourt, D. (2022). Patterns of compliance with COVID-19 preventive behaviours: A latent class analysis of 20 000 UK adults. *Journal of Epidemiology and Community Health*, *76*(3), 247–253.

5

LITERARY REPRESENTATIONS OF ILLNESS AND PUBLIC PERCEPTIONS

5.1 Introduction

You may wonder why a book on researching language and health includes a chapter on literary representations of illness. Let us begin with two extracts, both relevant to a mental health disorder known as schizophrenia. Example 5.1 is the definition of schizophrenia from the 5th edition of the *Diagnostic and Statistical Manual* – the most influential, as well as contested, guide to the diagnosis of mental illness:

EXAMPLE 5.1

The presence of 2 (or more) of the following, each present for a significant portion of time during a 1-month period (or less if successfully treated), with at least 1 of them being (1), (2), or (3): (1) delusions, (2) hallucinations, (3) disorganized speech, (4) grossly disorganized or catatonic behavior, and (5) negative symptoms.

(American Psychiatric Association 2013)

Example 5.2 is a passage from the book *Henry's Demons* (Cockburn & Cockburn, 2011), where Henry, a young man with a diagnosis of schizophrenia, gives an autobiographical account of one of several episodes in which he ran away from a psychiatric hospital:

EXAMPLE 5.2

I found myself walking on a road parallel to the train tracks. I felt I was going on a mission. You know fire hydrants are yellow and have an H on them. I thought the H stood for Henry. I climbed a barbed-wire fence and sat under a big tree. I put down all the stuff I had amassed: bits of metal, bits of wood, and

DOI: 10.4324/9781003020417-7

> a big bag of clay. I felt the tree telling me to take off my shoes. I was scared, as
> I had been arrested previously for not wearing shoes.
>
> *(Cockburn & Cockburn, 2011: 39–40)*

Although Henry does not accept the diagnosis of schizophrenia, the experience described in Extract 2 does fulfil some of the diagnostic criteria from Extract 1: he hears voices that other people cannot hear (hallucinations) and he believes things that others do not share, such as that the letter 'H' on a fire hydrant stands for his own name and that you can be arrested just for not wearing shoes (delusions). However, the two extracts contrast dramatically in terms of their perspective on schizophrenia. Extract 1 provides a technical, detached, third-person perspective, whereas Extract 2 provides a personal, involved, first-person perspective. This chapter focuses on the analysis of books such as *Henry's Demons* because the latter perspective is increasingly recognized as just as important as the first, both in clinical contexts and in the wider public perception of health and illness.

First-person narratives (including those shared in online environments – see Chapter 8) provide insights into the lived experience of illness and healthcare that are crucially important not just for understanding and empathy, but also for sensitive and effective diagnosis, support, and treatment. For example, a review of *Henry's Demons* from *The Guardian* newspaper emphasizes the depth of insight that can be reached by reading Henry's story:

> 'Can a man who is warm understand a man who is freezing?' Patrick Cockburn quotes Solzhenitsyn's question in the preface to this account of his son Henry's schizophrenia. The ensuing shared narrative brings the reader closer to such an understanding than anything else I've read.
>
> *(Charlotte Moore,* The Guardian, *26th February 2011)*

In addition, *Henry's Demons* has been reviewed in several medical journals (*The Lancet, Psychosis, The American Journal of Psychiatry*, and the *British Journal of Psychiatry*), where it is described, for example, as a 'must-read for anyone involved in treating individuals with schizophrenia' (Conlan, 2011: 434) and as 'a powerful illustration of what services stand to gain if they can learn from the experience and insights of patients and their families' (Bunker, 2012: 181).

This is not in fact unusual for autobiographies such as *Henry's Demons*, and also for novels whose protagonists are interpreted as having illnesses such as dementia or developmental conditions such as autism. Such published narratives can enable wide audiences to experience the internal perspective of individuals who have those particular experiences, including both challenges and, in some cases, additional insights. For example, Henry describes his own experiences as involving a 'spiritual awakening', and indeed readers of the book share his sense of wonder as well as his difficulties.

In this chapter we use the term 'literature' and 'literary' as umbrella terms for commercially published narrative accounts of illness and, in one case, conditions such as autism, whether they are presented as fiction (e.g. novels, films), non-fiction (autobiographies), or as lying somewhere between these two categories:

> Literature—both fiction in a range of forms and autobiographical narratives, including pathographies—can tell us not only about medicine or doctors, but also about the experience of health, sickness, illness, encounters with clinics and clinicians, the reactions of significant others, the support found in the strangest of places, the role and impact of informal caring, and the radical reordering necessary after the dramatic rift that significant illness causes through an individual life.
>
> *(Crawford et al., 2015: 38)*

Because they reach large numbers of both lay and professional audiences, these literary accounts influence perceptions and public debates, and are therefore worthy subjects for analysis, including the kind of linguistic analysis that is the concern of this book. This is evident in much recent work in Stylistics – the linguistic study of literature (Jeffries & McIntyre, 2010) – and in a growing tradition that applies insights from the humanities to the understanding and experience of health and illness, under the labels of Narrative Medicine (Charon, 2006), Medical Humanities (Bates et al., 2013) and Health Humanities (Crawford et al., 2015). We briefly return to the latter in Chapter 8.

5.1.1 In this chapter

The rest of this chapter is divided into two halves. First, we discuss the practical, methodological, and ethical considerations that are relevant to the analysis of literary representations of the experience of illness. Then we discuss a series of studies that involve different linguistic approaches to novels and autobiographies concerned with different illness experiences.

5.2 Preliminary considerations

In this section, we consider how the general methodological and ethical issues outlined in Chapters 2 and 3 apply to the study of literary representations of illness. Specifically, we discuss:

- Selecting a text or texts;
- Identifying the focus of your analysis;
- Managing long texts in small-case studies;
- Including interpretations other than your own;
- Ethics and copyright.

5.2.1 Selecting a text or texts

Let us begin with the selection of one or more texts for analysis. First, what should the text(s) be about? The suggestions we provide in Chapter 2 about choosing a specific illness or healthcare context to focus on apply here too. You may have personal reasons for being interested in, for example, narratives to do with depression, eating disorders, Long Covid, or being treated with chemotherapy for cancer. These personal reasons may be combined with external reasons as to why one or more narratives about that particular illness are worthy of investigation. For example, a particular novel or autobiography may have been published very recently; it may be a best-seller; it may have received one or more prestigious prizes; it may have sparked debates on social media or in the mainstream media; it may have been highlighted as valuable by a particular illness community, and/or it may belong to a genre or deal with a topic that has not received much attention before. Whichever combination of factors justify your decision, you will need to present them as clearly as possible when you are providing a rationale for your selection.

A common additional dilemma at the point of text selection is whether to analyze one or more texts. For example, should you study an individual narrative about the experience of anorexia, or should you study more than one and compare them? Both options are possible and justifiable in principle, as shown by the studies we discuss in this chapter. Focusing on a single text, with evidence of its personal, public, and scholarly relevance, is always a viable option, especially for a student project. For example, Harrison (2017) shows how the experience of dementia is represented in the best-selling 2014 novel *Elizabeth is Missing* by Emma Healey. Focusing on more than one text can be appropriate when there is a good reason to compare them and when the analysis is sufficiently focused to make this possible in the time and space available. For example, Emmott and Alexander (2016) show how similar linguistic devices are used to represent the experience of sudden physical disability (e.g. due to a stroke) in four different autobiographies. Generally speaking, however, it is seldom viable to conduct detailed qualitative analyses of more than three texts in a single student project or dissertation. A practical solution, early on in a project, to the dilemma about whether to analyze one text or several, is to begin to work on one text – the one you would not want to leave out of your study. After carrying out a preliminary analysis and beginning to draft your analysis sections, you will be in a better position to decide if there is time, space and a good rationale for carrying out the same analysis on one or more further texts.

5.2.2 Deciding on the focus of your analysis

Closely connected with decisions about text selection are decisions about the precise focus of your analysis. You may decide on a general focus, as reflected in a research question such as: *How is the experience of … represented in … ?* Harrison

(2017), for example, shows how, in the novel *Elizabeth is Missing*, the experience of dementia is conveyed through a range of different lexical, grammatical and narratological patterns. Or you may have a more specific focus in terms of the linguistic phenomenon/a you will investigate, which could be reflected in a question such as *How is metaphor used to convey the experience of … in … ?* For example, El Refaie (2019) shows how visual metaphors are used to convey particular aspects of the experiences of cancer and depression in contemporary graphic novels (see also Senkbeil & Hoppe, 2016 for a study of metaphors in an autobiographical account of eating disorders). Another way of narrowing your focus to allow for comparison is to select a topic for your analysis that involves analyzing small sections of longer narratives, such as looking at accounts of diagnosis in different narratives about the same illness. Other things being equal, a narrower focus is of course more appropriate when analyzing more than one text. However, Emmott and Alexander's (2016) study of the representation of acquired physical disability in four autobiographies is a good example of how to consider multiple linguistic devices in several texts within a single chapter-length study.

5.2.3 Managing long texts in small-scale studies

A methodological challenge that needs to be addressed when analyzing published literary narratives is how to manage book-length texts such as novels or other substantial works, such as feature films (and similar challenges exist when faced with large digital datasets, as in Chapters 7 and 8). Broadly speaking, there are three main options.

The first option is to make a principled selection of a series of extracts from the whole texts (usually no more than five) and analyze those in detail for the phenomenon/a that you set out to investigate. If you opt for this approach, you need a good rationale for selecting the extracts. For example, if you want to show change or progression in a narrative, you may choose an extract from the beginning, one from the middle and one from the end of the book, perhaps involving similar situations. If you are focusing on particular experiences, such as interactions with health professionals or accounts of hallucinations, you will select extracts that are concerned with those experiences. In all cases, extracts should be reasonably self-contained, for example in terms of a whole scene or episode in the narrative, and, for detailed analysis, should normally range between 500 and 1000 words each. For example, Harrison (2017) bases most of her analysis of *Elizabeth is Missing* on a substantial extract from the novel that concerns a particularly salient episode of the protagonist merging the past and the present in her mind.

The second option for dealing with lengthy texts applies where you are interested in very specific textual phenomena that may be scattered throughout the text, such as creative metaphors or the use of speech presentation or references to negative emotions. In this case, you would identify all relevant instances of the phenomenon in question as part of a systematic analysis to demonstrate the claims you want to make. The complete list of relevant examples could be placed in an appendix. For example, Emmott and Alexander (2016) state that, in the autobiographies they study, unusual, hyperbolic similes are used to convey the effort that routine activities require after being paralyzed by a stroke, and provide one or two examples each from the four narratives in question.

The third option is to employ corpus linguistic methods to analyze the complete text, possibly in combination with one of the first two options we have just described. For example, Demjén (2015) uses the corpus software Wmatrix to compare word frequencies in one of Sylvia Plath's diaries (the 'Smith journal') and a corpus of autobiographies. The results show that one of the keywords (see Chapter 2) in Plath's journal is the second-person pronoun 'you'. Demjén then observes that this is not just because of the use of 'you' in reports of dialogue, but because some entries in the journal are written in the second person, e.g.: '*There comes a time when* all your outlets are blocked, as with wax. You sit in your room, feeling the prickling ache in your body which constricts your throat, tightens dangerously in little tear pockets behind your eyes' (Demjén, 2015: 171). Further detailed analysis of second-person entries shows that they tend to involve 'firsts' (e.g. first time living away from home), that they involve emotional depth and tension, and that they cluster, for example, around Plath's suicide attempts. This leads to conclusions about second-person narration itself as well as the importance of attention to (second) pronoun usage in supporting and diagnosing people with mental health problems. Even without carrying out a corpus linguistic analysis, it is sometimes appropriate to provide some quantitative information in support of your claims, depending on what you want to show. We provide an example in relation to *Henry's Demons* later in this chapter.

5.2.4 Including interpretations other than your own

It is often useful to refer to existing responses to or interpretations of your text(s) as a springboard for your analysis or in support of your observations. In principle, it is possible to collect data on reader responses as part of your own study, for example via focus groups, questionnaires, or reading groups (e.g. Whiteley, 2020). This method involves gaining ethical approval, consent from participants, familiarity with the relevant data collection methods, and time and effort for the design of the response study and for the (transcription and) analysis of the resulting data. If you decide to go down this road, you need to be confident that you can handle all of this in the time you have.

There are also, however, other sources of data on how your chosen text has been received and interpreted by others. If your chosen text has been in the public domain sufficiently long, there may be literary critical studies about it. These provide professional readers' responses to texts and may also reflect particular scholarly perspectives in literary or cultural studies, based, for example, on feminism or Marxism or post-modernist theories. If your text is recent, there may not be a scholarly literature for you to refer to. However, you can search for and consider reviews by professional writers, such as journalists in the mainstream media, or by lay readers, for example on websites such as Amazon or Goodreads. These lay reviews can be cited as examples of how readers of the book have evaluated it and interpreted it, as evidence of trends and or disagreements in interpretation, or as raising questions that your analysis will help answer (e.g. Nuttall, 2018). If you make use of such sources, you can select and quote/summarize comments that are particularly relevant to your study or you can take a more systematic approach such as, for example, analyzing the main themes in the first 100 reviews on Goodreads, either manually or by means of corpus methods.

5.2.5 Ethics and copyright

The analysis of published texts does not require obtaining consent from the authors or permission to do the study, regardless of the sensitivity of the topic. Therefore, as we mentioned in Chapter 3, you may not have to submit an ethics application, or, if you are required to do so, you will not have any major issues to address. In the case of studies produced solely for the purpose of coursework or dissertations, there are usually no copyright issues involved in quoting from a published text. The UK, for example, makes an exception to copyright law for educational purposes. However, if you aim to publish your study, you need to check whether the text(s) you discuss are still under copyright and, if so, how much of the original text you are permitted to quote, or how many images you are permitted to reproduce, without submitting a request to the relevant copyright holders.

5.3 Selected studies

The rest of this chapter will provide you with concrete examples of linguistic analyses of literary representations of illness from different genres: novels, autobiographies and multimodal narratives. These studies mostly locate themselves within the interconnected fields of Stylistics – the linguistic study of literature (Jeffries & McIntyre, 2010), and Narratology – the academic study of narratives (Abbott, 2002). From the perspective of Narratology, Margolin (2003: 287) notes a 'preference of much literature for nonstandard forms of cognitive functioning, be they rare or marginal, deviant, or involving a failure, breakdown, or lack of standard patterns'. In practice, this often involves characters who are interpreted as having a particular illness or being affected by some form of disability. In Stylistics, the notion of 'mind style', i.e. 'any distinctive linguistic representation of an individual mental self' (Fowler, 1977: 103), is similarly applied to how novels in particular convey characters' experience of mental of physical illness (e.g. Semino & Swindlehurst, 1996, Emmott & Alexander, 2016, Demjén & Semino, 2021). Both traditions also emphasize how experiencing minds – and bodies – that work in unusual ways can enable readers to reassess what it means to be 'healthy' or 'normal'. As Margolin puts it:

> [t]he fictional presentation of cognitive mechanisms in action, especially of their own breakdown and failure, is itself a powerful cognitive tool which may make us aware of actual cognitive mechanisms, and, more specifically, of our own mental functioning.
>
> *(Margolin, 2003: 278)*

A wide range of linguistic or textual phenomena can be involved in conveying 'cognitive function' or 'mind style' in literature. The studies we have selected in this and the next section will give you a good idea of that range, by focusing in turn on speech presentation, narrative structure, foregrounding devices, cognitive grammar and text worlds, the pragmatics of interaction, and visual metaphors. Throughout, we also point out how different scholars have made the decisions and addressed the methodological challenges and issues we mentioned in the previous section.

5.3.1 Representing aspects of mental illness in autobiography

Let us go back to the book *Henry's Demons*, which we mentioned in the Introduction. *Henry's Demons* is a multi-voiced autobiography as it alternates between first-person accounts from three people: Henry Cockburn, who was diagnosed with schizophrenia in 2002 at the age of 20, after a series of psychotic episodes; Henry's father Patrick, who is a journalist and writer; and, in a small section of the book, Henry's mother Jan Montefiore, a professor of English. While the multi-voiced nature of the book provides different perspectives on Henry's difficulties, diagnosis, repeated hospitalizations, and multiple escapes from hospitals, the most relevant sections of the book for our purposes are those written by Henry himself.

Two studies by two of the current authors (ES and ZD) have focused on several different aspects of Henry's narrative, to show what a linguistic analysis can reveal about his experiences, as well as to account for the success of the book and its potential to generate understanding and empathy for Henry and people who may have similar experiences.

Demjén and Semino (2015) combine detailed textual analyses with the quantification of selected linguistic patterns to study systematically the extracts from Henry's chapter (49 in total) in which he represents the experience of hearing voices that other people cannot hear, also known as Auditory Verbal Hallucinations. They do this by drawing from a particularly relevant contribution from Stylistics: the development of typologies of speech presentation, which capture the different ways in which others' words can be reported, and the implications of different choices (e.g. Leech & Short, 1981). A central distinction here is between Direct Speech presentation, which is conventionally associated with the verbatim reproduction of utterances, and several non-direct forms, the best known of which is Indirect Speech presentation. For example, in Example 5.3 below, the use of quotation marks and the first-person plural 'we' are typical of Direct Speech presentation, and give the impression that Henry is reproducing word by word what the voices said:

EXAMPLE 5.3

> I remember the brambles saying, 'We are the gods.'
>
> *(Cockburn & Cockburn, 2011: 87)*

In contrast, Example 5.4 is a case of Indirect Speech presentation, where Henry as narrator provides the content of what the leaves said to him, using words that reflect his perspective (e.g. 'me' and 'my' where the voices would use 'you' and 'your'):

EXAMPLE 5.4

> I thought the leaves of ivy brushing against my skin were telling me to pull down my trousers.
>
> *(Cockburn & Cockburn, 2011: 89)*

A striking feature of Henry's narrative is that he only uses Direct Speech for voices that others cannot hear in 7 out of 49 cases, i.e. approximately 14% of cases. In all other cases he uses Indirect Speech or other forms of speech presentation (Semino & Short, 2014) that do not claim to be verbatim reports (e.g. 'There is a tree I sit under in the garden in Lewisham which speaks to me and gives me hope'; p. 222). This, Demjén and Semino (2015) discover, contrasts with how Henry reports voices that other people can also hear, where he uses Direct Speech around 40% of the time. This is close to what has been found to be the average incidence of Direct Speech in autobiographical narratives generally (Semino & Short, 2014).

In addition Demjén and Semino point out some distinctive patterns in Henry's choice of verbs used to introduce utterances attributed to hallucinatory voices:

EXAMPLE 5.5

> I felt the tree telling me to take off my shoes.
>
> *(Cockburn & Cockburn, 2011: 39)*

EXAMPLE 5.6

> I could feel it [the root of a tree] talking to me in my head.
>
> *(Cockburn & Cockburn, 2011: 39)*

EXAMPLE 5.7

> I felt a call from the natural world to run away […].
>
> *(Cockburn & Cockburn, 2011: 217)*

The verb 'feel' is an unusual choice of verb to precede speech-related verbs such as 'tell', because it relates to the sensory experience of touch rather than sound. The combination of a low frequency of Direct Speech presentation and the use of non-auditory verbs such as 'feel' can be interpreted as a reflection of Henry's own experiences of different kinds of voices. The voices that other people cannot hear seem to lend themselves less naturally to verbatim representations, and to involve senses other than hearing. This confirms and further deepens what is known about the phenomenology, or lived experience, of voice hearing, namely that it may be different from hearing voices that others can also hear. This may be partly disguised by the term 'voice hearing' itself and by the lack of words that capture what Henry seems to be suggesting: the process of receiving messages, meanings or communication without associated sounds, and, in some cases, through his whole body rather than his ears.

Another distinctive aspect of Henry's chapters is his approach to storytelling. Example 5.8 below is discussed in Demjén and Semino (2021):

EXAMPLE 5.8

> We sat on the bank of the river playing Bob Marley, and I felt a force pulling me into the Thames, but I resisted it and didn't jump in. The tide was going out and we went down some stairs and sat on a stretch of sand. A nice woman said there was going to be a concert on the sand later, and I saw the water lapping on the shore. I said, 'Move back, move back, sea.' A man whom I think was dealing heroin shouted 'Fuck off' at me. We walked to a place where there were skateboarders, and I saw a red bus crossing the Thames and felt I should have been on that bus. A girl with a Russian accent asked to take a picture of us, and again I felt paranoid. We were in Charing Cross, and everybody seemed to be looking at us, and I pulled a stupid face when she took the picture.
>
> *(Cockburn & Cockburn, 2011: 192–3)*

On the one hand, this extract has some clear characteristics of an episode of narrative. It tells of a series of events which appear to be in chronological order, and it involves human participants engaged in different activities, including some verbal interaction. On the other hand, however, there is no obvious cause–effect relationship between the different events, and no continuity in terms of characters other than the presence of Henry himself. In the terms used in psychiatry for the symptoms of schizophrenia, this could be evidence of 'deficits in coherence' and 'looseness of associations' (e.g. Marini et al., 2008; Perlini et al., 2012).

From a linguistic and narratological perspective, however, Demjén and Semino account both for what is unusual and what is meaningful and even somewhat familiar about Henry's storytelling. The passage is unlike the relatively formal written kind of storytelling associated with autobiographies, for the reasons we just mentioned: lack of clear cause–effect relationships between events and lack of persistence of characters. On the other hand, the passage is in some ways reminiscent of the 'small stories' (Georgakopoulou, 2007) that we may find in more informal contexts, and of the mostly fictional narratives that revolve around a character's 'experientiality' (Fludernik, 1996) rather than on conventional plot development. These observations account both for what may be perceived as peculiar or distinctive about Henry's style of storytelling and for the fact that it is still both comprehensible and poignant. It reveals how Henry perceives the world, and the people and events within it, as a series of intense and sometimes disconcerting moments, which can both fascinate him and, at times, overwhelm him.

We mentioned earlier that the study of published autobiographies such as *Henry's Demons* does not require the consent of the authors, nor ethics clearance. This does not mean, however, that such studies can completely disregard the potential consequences of the research for the authors, especially when they are in a vulnerable situation. The two co-authors of the present book that studied *Henry's Demons* ensured that the Cockburn family were aware of the research and had a chance to comment, if they so wished. More importantly, Henry was considered in those studies as an 'expert by experience' in voice hearing and psychosis, and his view that his experiences were not a symptom of a mental illness, let alone schizophrenia, were presented alongside the fact that those very experiences resulted in a diagnosis of schizophrenia.

5.3.2 *Representing physical and cognitive decline in fiction and non-fiction*

In contrast to Demjén and Semino's analyses of a single text, Emmott and Alexander (2016) apply some core concepts in Stylistics to what they describe as four 'medical autobiographies of literary quality' (Emmott & Alexander, 2016: 289): Jean-Dominique Bauby's (2008) *The Diving-Bell and the Butterfly*, Robert McCrum's (1998) *My Year Off: Rediscovering Life After a Stroke*; Jane Lapotaire's (2004) *Time out of Mind*; and Ulla-Carin Lindquist's (2005) *Rowing without Oars*. All four authors started their lives as healthy and able-bodied, and were eventually physically disabled or almost completely paralyzed in their 40s or 50s, due to sudden or progressive neurological illness: a stroke for Bauby and McCrum, a brain haemorrhage due to an aneurysm for Lapotaire and ALS (Amyotrophic Lateral Sclerosis) for Lindquist. McCrum and Lapotaire narrate their slow recoveries, while Bauby and Lindquist died about a year after the onset of the neurological illness they talk about in their stories.

Emmott and Alexander focus their analysis on different kinds of relevant effects or themes, such as 'Disorientation' and 'Adjusting to illness and disability', which they see as corresponding to different aspects of each author's mind style. In each section of the analysis, Emmott and Alexander show how all four books employ similar devices to convey what it is like to suddenly lose control of one's body, to attempt to recover or slow down one's deterioration, but, most of all, to experience one's own body, identity, and life in a dramatically different way. Emmott and Alexander quote many extracts from each text to show how these effects are achieved via linguistic choices and patterns that share some element of 'deviation' from expectations, such as sentence fragments (Example 5.9), hyperbolic figurative comparisons (Example 5.10) and unusual personifications (Example 5.11).

EXAMPLE 5.9

Someone must have taken [my hearing aid] out of my ear when … when … when what? When. I. Fell.

(Lapoitaire, 2004: 20)

EXAMPLE 5.10

A very black fly settles on my nose. I waggle my head to unseat him. Olympic wrestling is child's play compared to this.

(Bauby, 2008: 110)

EXAMPLE 5.11

I feel satisfied when I drive away from there. So does my hand, as it lies in its cradle

(Lindquist, 2005: 25)

Drawing from Stylistics, Emmott and Alexander point out how these different linguistic choices function as foregrounding devices (Leech, 1969, Short, 1996): they draw readers' attention to the relevant stretches of text and the experiences they convey. More specifically, these foregroundings facilitate the experience of 'defamiliarization' (Šklovsky, 2012/1965) by portraying familiar experiences in unfamiliar ways. Neurological illness forces each author to experience the world in new, alien ways, and their narratives enable the reader to share those fresh and deeply challenging perspectives.

In Example 5.9, the use of one-word sentences for what would more normally be a single sentence ('When. I. Fell') may 'iconically reflect the difficulty of articulating the key point of collapse' (Emmott & Alexander, 2016: 293). The hyperbolic figurative comparison in Example 5.10 (between slightly moving one's head and Olympic wrestling) conveys the enormous effort and sense of achievement that minimal movements can involve after a stroke. And the attribution of an evaluative attitude to the narrator's hand (as opposed to 'I') in Example 5.11 suggests that the author no longer perceives her own body as a single coherent whole that she has control over.

Emmott and Alexander's analyses also show different nuances of defamiliarization. On the one hand, the use of the various foregrounding devices suggests trauma, disorientation, a disruption in one's personal and social identities, and a sense of estrangement from one's own body. On the other hand, an intense focus on the minute details of one's own body and surroundings, which were previously taken for granted, leads to a deeper appreciation of life, both as it was and as it currently is. Lindquist, for example, is quoted as commenting that 'Death brings me closer to life' and 'I would not wish to be without this part of my life' (Emmott & Alexander, 2016: 304).

A different stylistic study of mind style applies some aspects of cognitive grammar (Langacker, 2008) and text world theory (Werth, 1999) to a single fictional text: Emma Healey's 2014 novel *Elizabeth is Missing* (Harrison, 2017). The novel is narrated by Maud, a woman in her 80s who, readers are likely to infer, has dementia. As Harrison points out, it shares some of the features of detective fiction, as it involves parallels between Maud's current effort to find her friend Elizabeth and the disappearance of her own sister, Sukey, 70 years previously. Harrison's analysis shows how different aspects of the narrative convey Maud's experience of dementia, including her inability to remember the names of everyday objects and to separate her present-day experiences from her memories of the past.

This is, for example, how Maud refers to, respectively, a toaster and a packet of pencils:

EXAMPLE 5.12

bread-heater, the bread browner

(Healey, 2014: 82)

EXAMPLE 5.13

a packet of lamp posts, tiny lamp posts with lead through the middle
(Healey, 2014: 217) (Harrison, 2017: 142)

Drawing from cognitive grammar, Harrison describes these examples as instances of 'overspecification', whereby Maud 'relies on descriptions of an object's schematic properties' to compensate for a memory gap (Harrison, 2017: 142–3). More broadly, these descriptions simultaneously convey the challenges that Maud experiences and her creativity and determination in expressing herself. As such, like the rest of the novel, they are simultaneously sad and humorous.

Harrison's argument about how Maud's dementia is conveyed in the novel is primarily based on a detailed analysis of an extract of approximately 500 words. In the extract, Maud and her daughter Helen are having lunch in a restaurant. During the meal, Helen becomes frustrated by her mother's forgetfulness, to which Maud reacts with an outburst of anger:

EXAMPLE 5.14

I don't answer; my teeth are still tight together. I feel I might start screaming, but breaking something, that's a good idea. That's exactly what I want to do. I pick up my butter knife and stab it into the black side plate. The china breaks. Helen says something, swearing I think, and somebody rushes towards me. I keep looking at the plate. The middle has crumbled slightly and it looks like a broken record, a broken gramophone record.

I found some once in our back garden. They were in the vegetable patch, smashed to bits and jumbled together. Ma had sent me out to help Dad when I'd got back from school and he'd handed me his shovel for digging a runner-bean trench, before disappearing into the shed. The records were almost the same colour as the soil and I wouldn't have found them, only I felt something snap as I dug and a few moments later the shards caught between the prongs of my fork […]

It didn't take me long to connect the pieces, and it was nice work in the winter sun, listening to the music of the pigeons as they cooed to one another. It was like doing a jigsaw puzzle, except that even when I'd finished there were still some bits missing. I could read the labels now, though: 'Virginia', 'We Three' and 'I'm Nobody's Baby'.

I sat back on my heels. These were my sister's favourites, the ones she always asked Douglas to play. And now here they were, smashed up and buried amongst the remains of rhubarb and onions.

(Healey, 2014: 19–21)

Harrison points out that this extract involves two different 'text worlds', defined as settings located in particular places and times, and including particular characters and objects: the current scene in the restaurant (text world 1) and a scene in the past where, shortly after her sister's disappearance, Maud unearths in the garden of her youth some records that belonged to her (text world 2). The sight of the broken plate in text world 1 triggers the memory that constitutes text world 2, based on a visual similarity: the presence of objects that are round, black and broken. In Harrison's cognitive linguistic terms, the plate/records pair is a 'narrative anchor' that connects the two text worlds. However, the lack of an explicit transition to that earlier time (note 'I found some in our back garden' at the beginning of the second paragraph) suggests that past and present merge in Maud's mind.

Harrison suggests that the extract she has selected for detailed analysis displays the key features of Maud's narrative that readers are likely to interpret as evidence of her dementia. Maud's memories of the past are preserved, while the present often escapes from her mental grasp. As a consequence of that, she relies on the past to make sense of the present, for example in assuming that Elizabeth is missing in the same way as Suky once was. The text world approach is also particularly suitable to account for the role and connections between past and present in the novel, which are particularly important given the association between dementia and memory problems. We will briefly return to Harrison's study at the end of the next section.

5.3.3 Interactional patterns and autism-spectrum disorder in three novels

Our final example in this section is a study by one of the current authors of how conversations within a novel can suggest that a character has an autism-spectrum disorder (Semino, 2014). Autism involves a diagnostic process but is not an illness, of course. From a clinical perspective, it is usually defined as a developmental disorder whereby some people have difficulties with communication, socialization, and imagination (e.g. Baron-Cohen, 1995: 60). From the perspective of the neurodiversity paradigm, in contrast, it is described as a particular way of seeing and experiencing the world – no less valid or healthy than the perspectives of people who may be described as 'neurotypical'. We include this study here, however, for two reasons. First, literary representations of autism, whether fictional or non-fictional, are often similar in their motivation and cultural influence as published narratives about illness: they provide first-person accounts of the phenomenology of experiences that are not always well understood, and, by doing so, they can provide validation or opportunities for empathy and greater understanding. Second, the kind of analysis demonstrated in this study shows how, as mentioned in Chapter 2, linguistic frameworks that were developed for the analysis of 'real life' interactions are potentially relevant to the analysis of reports of conversations in illness narratives where the protagonist finds communication or interaction challenging in some way.

In the extract below (which we briefly introduced in Chapter 1), Christopher, the narrator/protagonist of Mark Haddon *The Curious Incident of the Dog in the Night-Time* (2003), is being questioned by a policeman after being found holding the corpse of his next-door neighbour's dog, who has a garden fork sticking out of its stomach:

EXAMPLE 5.15

> The policeman squatted down beside me and said, 'Would you like to tell me what's going on here, young man?'
> I sat up and said, 'The dog is dead.'
> 'I'd got that far,' he said.
> I said, 'I think someone killed the dog.'
> 'How old are you?' he asked.
> I replied, 'I am 15 years and 3 months and 2 days.' (Haddon, 2003: 7)

Semino (2014) uses Grice's Cooperative Principle (1989) and its subsequent developments to describe the conversation, and its implications for attributing to Christopher an autism-spectrum disorder. In Grice's terms, Christopher breaks one of the 'maxims' that underlie cooperative communicative behaviour, the Maxim of Quantity:

> The category of Quantity relates to the quantity of information to be provided, and under it fall the following maxims:

1. Make your contribution as informative as is required (for the current purposes of the exchange).
2. Do not make your contribution more informative than is required. (Grice, 1989: 26.)

Christopher's first two answers to the policeman's questions are not as informative as required, as it is obvious not just that the dog is dead, but that it has been killed. Indeed, that is why the police have been called in the first place. In contrast, Christopher's third answer is more informative than is required, as specifying months and days with regard to age is very unusual, beyond babyhood and some specific medical settings. When Grice's maxims are intentionally broken, the speaker may be attempting to deceive the interlocutor, or to convey implicit meanings. Here, however, readers are likely to conclude that Christopher had no such intentions: he 'infringes' the Maxim of quantity, i.e. he breaks it inadvertently, while in fact trying to be helpful (Thomas, 1995). Attributing to Christopher an autism-spectrum disorder is one way of explaining this infringement. This is because one of the characteristics that are associated with autism-spectrum disorders is difficulties with 'reading' others' minds, i.e. attributing beliefs and emotions to others. In Christopher's case, this involves understanding what the policeman is likely to know already and what new information he requires (e.g. Baron-Cohen, 1995).

Semino shows how similar conversational episodes occur in two other contemporary novels that, unlike *The Curious Incident*, mention autism-spectrum disorders explicitly: *The Speed of Dark* by Elizabeth Moon (2002) and *The Language of Others* by Clare Morrall (2008).

The extract below from *The Speed of Dark*, involves Lou, who says he has autism, and Mr Crenshaw, Lou's new line manager at a company that employs people with autism for jobs that require an exceptional sensitivity to patterns.

EXAMPLE 5.16

Mr Crenshaw comes up again at closing time, when I am still working. He opens my door without knocking. I don't know how long he was there before I noticed him, but I am sure he did not knock. I jump when he says 'Lou!' and turn around.

'What are you doing?' he asks.

'Working,' I say. What did he think? What else could I be doing in my office, at my workstation? (Moon, 2002: 25)

In *The Language of Others*, the protagonist, Jessica, is also sometimes flummoxed by other people's questions. In the extract below, her new boyfriend is being shown around Jessica's family home, a large but dilapidated stately home:

EXAMPLE 5.17

'So which bit do you live in?'

   I couldn't decide what he meant. Was he talking about me personally? My bedroom? Or which bit did we all live in? What did he mean by 'live'? The kitchen? Or the drawing room? I didn't know how to answer.

   'We live in all of it,' said my father.

   'Really?' said Andrew. 'Wow.'

(Morrall, 2008: 24)

As these extracts show, all three protagonists sometimes find it difficult to understand precisely what other characters mean through some of their utterances and, as a consequence, sometimes provide answers that can be misinterpreted as flippant, as in Christopher's and Lou's case, or no response at all, as in Jessica's case. Similarly, Semino shows that all three characters sometimes cause accidental offence by telling the truth (i.e. complying with Grice's Maxim of Quality) even when that involves an unnecessary threat to another character's face (Brown & Levinson, 1987). Both patterns of behaviour can be explained by attributing to each character some difficulties with mind reading, and hence contribute to the projection of mind styles associated with autism-spectrum disorders.

   Both Harrison and Semino recognize that the novels they analyze should not be expected, never mind intended, to be medically correct. However, they point out that such novels nonetheless reflect and reinforce public perceptions of different illnesses or conditions, and are therefore particularly worthy of detailed investigation, including by asking how they relate to the experiences of 'real' people. On the one hand, fictional representations such as these can reinforce stereotypes (e.g. the idea that people with autism are also savants, which applies, at least to some extent, to both Christopher and Lou) or increase stigma (e.g. the idea that people with dementia are 'victims' of the illness and cannot live meaningful, fulfilling lives). On the other hand, these narratives can provide opportunities for increased empathy and understanding, and also for questioning what it means to be 'normal'. For example, the questions that the three protagonists find hard to understand are indeed, if one stops to look at them, rather vague (e.g. 'what's going on here?'). And the reason why all three characters sometimes cause offence is because they tell what they believe to be true even when it may be socially disadvantageous. Like Emmott and Alexander (2016), Semino (2014) uses the concept of defamiliarization to capture the potential that the three novels have to encourage readers to look differently at themselves and at communication and relationships around them, regardless of where they are positioned in relation to what counts as 'normal' in their societies.

5.3.4 Multimodal representations of depression and cancer in graphic novels

The types of texts we have discussed so far in this chapter are 'monomodal' texts – they rely on one single mode of communication: the (written) word. We now turn to studies that focus on multimodal narratives of illness, showing what effects can be achieved by combining the (written) word with visual images. We extend our discussion of multimodality in Chapter 4 by focusing on a study involving visual metaphors.

Figure 5.1 is an illustration from *My Depression: A Picture Book* by Elizabeth Swados, one of 35 graphic illness narratives analyzed in El Refaie's (2019) book *Visual Metaphor and Embodiment in Graphic Illness Narratives*.

This illustration shows the protagonist of the story standing behind prison bars in an inset placed in the middle of a clock hanging from a wall. The sentence 'Each moment feels like it lasts forever' is placed just below the clock. El Refaie points out that the positioning of the protagonist behind prison bars is consistent with conventional metaphors of depression as containment in an enclosed space

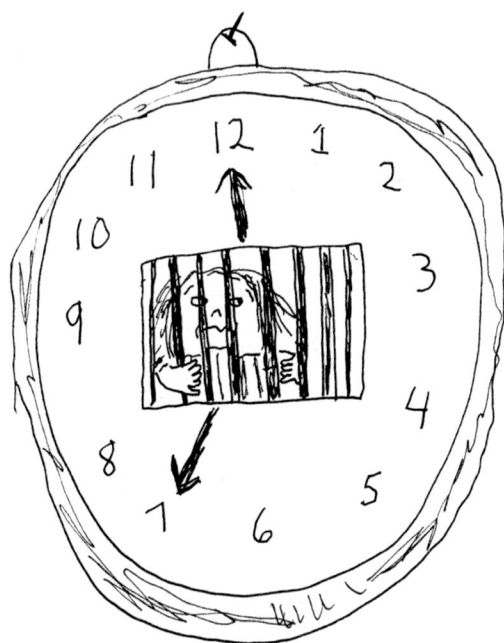

Each moment feels like it lasts forever.

FIGURE 5.1   From My Depression: A Picture Book by Elizabeth Swados (2005) © 2005 Elizabeth Swados

or entrapment, which had been previously identified in, for example, Sylvia Plath's diaries (Demjén, 2011, 2015) and interviews with people with depression (Charteris-Black, 2012). In previous studies, however, such Containment metaphors for depression had been linked to the LIFE IS A JOURNEY metaphor, within which the inability to move prevents people from achieving their life goals. In Figure 5.1, however, a visual metaphor of depression as entrapment is combined with references to the experience of temporality – metonymically via the clock (i.e. via an association between a time-keeping device and time itself) and explicitly in the caption. The combination of text and image therefore suggests that, as a consequence of depression, time is not felt to 'pass' in the normal way, so that the person feels that they are constantly experiencing an unpleasant, unchanging present. This is part of a pattern that El Refaie identifies in several different graphic novels about depression, out of a set of eight included in her study:

> When examining my corpus of graphic illness narratives about depression, however, I have discovered such a close link between the notions of spatial and temporal containment that I propose considering the experience that is being conveyed as a form of entrapment in spacetime.
>
> *(El Refaie, 2019: 180)*

Similarly, El Refaie identifies a distinctive pattern in the visual metaphors used in graphic narratives about cancer, whereby the experience of cancer is associated with distorted vision. For example, in Ball's *Inflatable Woman*, an illustration depicting the protagonist's experience of a mammography (Figure 5.2) shows a tilted mammograph machine and an incongruous imbalance in size between the protagonist herself and the nurse conducting the mammography: the protagonist is unusually small, for an adult, compared with the nurse. These features of the image, combined with the illegible marks in the nurse's speech bubble, convey the protagonist's 'terror and confusion' (El Refaie, 2019: 151). Above the whole scene, a giant eye suggests the presence of a doctor who will soon look at the scans and diagnose the protagonist's breast cancer. A quote from Robert Louis Stevenson's poem 'The sick child' is arranged in the top right corner in such a way as to associate the word 'God' with the doctor's seemingly all-seeing eye.

Based on an analysis of ten graphic narratives about cancer, El Refaie connects these visual metaphors to the centrality of 'seeing' and 'not seeing' in relation to this particular illness. On the one hand, both the illness and the treatment can cause major visible physical changes in the person who is sick. On the other hand, most tumours are invisible to the naked eye and can only be revealed by means of medical technology. El Refaie suggests that this challenges the conventional conceptual metaphor KNOWING IS SEEING:

> many of the visual metaphors in graphic illness narratives about cancer unsettle the connections between seeing and knowing that are so deeply

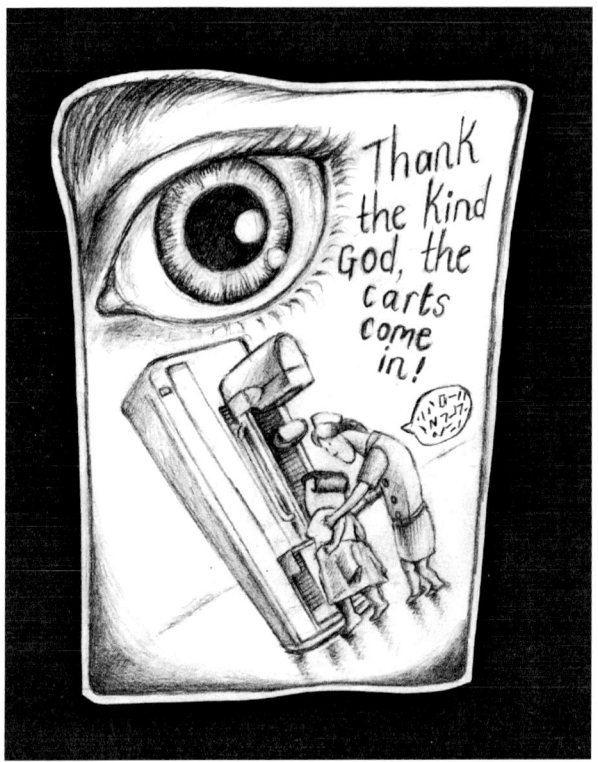

FIGURE 5.2 From The Inflatable Woman by Rachael Ball (2015) © 2015 Rachel Ball

entrenched in western culture in general and in contemporary western medicine in particular.

(El Refaie, 2019: 153)

El Refaie (2019: 11) describes her dataset as consisting of '35 graphic illness narratives (or "graphic pathographies") by North American and European authors on a range of physical and mental diseases', with the majority dealing with cancer or mood disorders. Most of the texts are described as memoirs, i.e. as autobiographical narratives about the author's own experiences (whether as a patient or as a carer), while a few are fictional. However, the visual nature of the genre arguably blurs the boundary between the fictional and the non-fictional, as authors have to create visual counterparts of themselves and other characters.

Among other things, El Refaie's detailed qualitative analyses of selected examples are used to challenge the view of the body that is prevalent in theories of metaphor and embodiment, namely as a shared, accessible, relatively stable part of our experience, which mostly functions as the source domain of metaphors. El Refaie points out how our experience of our own bodies is in fact dynamic, unstable and transient, and that graphic narratives are particularly well suited to convey the ways in which serious illness destabilizes and problematizes our perceptions of our own bodies (see also Emmott & Alexander, 2016). In the data she analyzes, the body itself tends to function as the target domain of a range of metaphors for the consequences of illness and for how we attempt to make sense of it.

5.4 Concluding remarks

This chapter has focused on literary representations of illness, because, whether fictional or non-fictional, they can provide important insights into the lived experience of illness, and contribute to public perceptions and debates. Drawing from Stylistics and related areas, we have shown how a range of linguistic as well as visual phenomena are relevant to literary representations of the experience of illness, including speech presentation, narrative structure, foregrounding devices, cognitive grammar and text worlds, the pragmatics of interaction, and multimodal metaphors.

Further readings

Ensslin, A. (2012). 'I want to say I may have seen my son die this morning': Unintentional unreliable narration in digital fiction. *Language and Literature, 21*(2), 136–149.

Lugea, J. (2022). Dementia mind styles in contemporary narrative fiction. *Language and Literature, 31*(2), 168–195.

Senkbeil, K., & Hoppe, N. (2016). 'The sickness stands at your shoulder …': Embodiment and cognitive metaphor in Hornbacher's wasted: A memoir of anorexia and bulimia. *Language and Literature, 25*(1), 3–17.

Whiteley, S. (2020). Interpreting (autistic?) mind style. *Anglistik, 31*(1), 71–89.

References

Abbott, H. P. (2002). *The Cambridge introduction to narrative*. Cambridge University Press.

American Psychiatric Association. (2013). *Diagnostic and statistical manual of mental disorders: DSM-5* (5th ed.). American Psychiatric Publishing.

Ball, R. (2015). *The inflatable woman*. Bloomsbury.

Baron-Cohen, S. (1995). *Mindblindness: An essay on autism and theory of mind*. MIT Press.

Bates, V., Bleakley, A., & Goodman, S. (2013). *Medicine, health and the arts: Approaches to the medical humanities*. Taylor & Francis.

Bauby, J.-D. (2008). *The diving-bell and the butterfly*. Harper Perennial.

Brown, P., & Levinson, S. C. (1987). *Politeness: Some universals in language use*. Cambridge University Press.

Bunker, N. (2012). Henry's demons: Living with schizophrenia. *Psychosis, 4*(2), 180–181.

Charon, R. (2006). *Narrative medicine: Honoring the stories of illness*. Oxford University Press.

Charteris-Black, J. (2012). Shattering the bell jar: Metaphor, gender, and depression. *Metaphor and Symbol*, *27*(3), 199–216.

Cockburn, P., & Cockburn, H. (2011). *Henry's demons*. Simon & Schuster.

Conlan, L. (2011). Henry's demons: Living with schizophrenia, a father and Son's story by Patrick and H. Cockburn. *British Journal of Psychiatry*, *199*(5), 434–434.

Crawford, P., Brown, B., & Baker, C. (2015). *Health humanities*. Palgrave Macmillan.

Demjen, Z. (2011). Motion and conflicted self metaphors in Sylvia Plath's 'Smith Journal'. *Metaphor and the Social World*, *1*(1), 7–25.

Demjen, Z. (2015). *Sylvia Plath and the language of affective states written discourse and the experience of depression*. Bloomsbury.

Demjén, Z., & Semino, E. (2015). Henry's voices: The representation of auditory verbal hallucinations in an autobiographical narrative. *BMJ Medical Humanities*, *41*(1), 57–62.

Demjén, Z., & Semino, E. (2021). Stylistics: Mind style in an autobiographical account of schizophrenia. In G. Brookes & D. Hunt (Eds.), *Analysing health communication: Discourse approaches* (pp. 333–356). Palgrave.

El Refaie, E. (2019). *Visual metaphor and embodiment in graphic illness narratives*. Oxford University Press.

Emmott, C., & Alexander, M. (2016). Defamiliarisation and foregrounding: Representing experiences of change of state and perception in neurological illness autobiographies. In V. Sotirova (Ed.), *The Bloomsbury companion to stylistics*, Series: Bloomsbury companions (pp. 289–307). Bloomsbury.

Fludernik, M. (1996). *Towards a 'natural' Narratology*. Routledge.

Fowler, R. (1977). *Linguistics and the novel*. Methuen.

Georgakopoulou, A. (2007). *Small stories, interaction and identities*. John Benjamins.

Grice, H. P. (1989). *Studies in the way of words*. Harvard University Press.

Haddon, M. (2003). *The curious incident of the dog in the night-time*. Jonathan Cape.

Harrison, C. (2017). Finding Elizabeth: Construing memory in Elizabeth is missing by Emma Healey. *Journal of Literary Semantics*, *46*(2), 131–151.

Healey, E. (2014). *Elizabeth is missing*. Harper Collins.

Jeffries, L., & McIntyre, D. (2010). *Stylistics*. Cambridge University Press.

Langacker, R. (2008). *Cognitive grammar*. Oxford University Press.

Lapotaire, J. (2004). *Time out of mind*. Virago.

Leech, G. (1969). *A linguistic guide to English poetry*. Longman.

Leech, G. N., & Short, M. H. (1981). *Style in fiction*. Longman.

Lindquist, U.-C. (2005). *Rowing without oars*. John Murray.

Margolin, U. (2003). Cognitive science, the thinking mind, and literary narrative. In D. Herman (Ed.), *Narrative theory and the cognitive sciences* (pp. 271–294). Center for the Study of Language and Information.

Marini, A., Spoletini, I., Rubino, I. A., Ciuffa, M., Bria, P., Martinotti, G., Banfi, G., Boccascino, R., Perla, S., Siracusano, A., Caltagirone, C. and Spalletta, G. (2008). The language of schizophrenia: An analysis of micro and macrolinguistic abilities and their neuro- psychological correlates. *Schizophrenia Research*, *105*(1–3), 144–155.

McCrum, R. (1998). *My year off: Rediscovering life after a stroke*. Picador.

Moon, E. (2002). *Speed of dark*. Orbit.

Moore, C. (2011). Henry's demons by Patrick and H Cockburn: Review. *The Guardian Newspaper*. Retrieved October 8, 2022, from https://www.theguardian.com/books/2011/feb/26/henrys-demons-patrick-henry-cockburn

Morrall, C. (2008). *The language of others*. Sceptre.

Nuttall, L. (2018). *Mind style and cognitive grammar: Language and worldview in speculative fiction.* Bloomsbury.

Perlini, C., Marini, A., Garzitto, M., Isola, M., Cerruti, S., Marinelli, V., Rambaldelli, G., Ferro, A., Tomelleri, L., Dusi, N., Bellani, N., Tansella, M., Fabbro, F. and Brambilla, P. (2012). Linguistic production and syntactic comprehension in schizophrenia and bipolar disorder. *Acta Psychiatrica Scandinavica, 126*(5), 363–376.

Šklovsky, V. (2012/1965). Art as technique. In L. T. Lemon & M. J. Reis (Eds.), *Russian formalism: Four essays* (pp. 3–24). University of Nebraska Press.

Semino, E. (2014). Pragmatic failure, mind style and characterization in fiction about autism. *Language and Literature, 23*(2), 141–158.

Semino, E., & Short, M. (2014). *Corpus stylistics: Speech, writing and thought presentation in a corpus of English writing.* Routledge.

Semino, E., & Swindlehurst, K. (1996). Metaphor and mind style in Ken Kesey's one flew over the cuckoo's nest. *Style, 30*(1), 143–166.

Senkbeil, K., & Hoppe, N. (2016). 'The sickness stands at your shoulder …': Embodiment and cognitive metaphor in Hornbacher's wasted: A memoir of anorexia and bulimia. *Language and Literature, 25*(1), 3–17.

Short, M. (1996). *Exploring the language of poems, plays and prose.* Longman.

Thomas, J. (1995). *Meaning in interaction.* Longman.

Werth, P. (1999). *Text worlds: Representing conceptual space in discourse.* Longman.

6

NEGOTIATING RELATIONSHIPS AND IDENTITIES IN SPOKEN HEALTHCARE INTERACTIONS

6.1 Introduction

Spoken interaction is a crucial way in which the day-to-day work of healthcare is done and an important research area in language and health. Millions of spoken interactions take place in healthcare settings each day, from consultations between patients and primary care providers to discussions between professionals in healthcare teams. It is an area where social relationships, such as those between doctors and patients, are important, particularly since people with everyday lived experiences of health and illness come into contact with the authoritative medical expertise of healthcare – what Mishler (1984: 14) differentiated as the 'voice of the lifeworld' and the 'voice of medicine'. The actions performed in these encounters are done through talk, such as a patient presenting their history, a healthcare professional delivering a diagnosis or the joint negotiation of a treatment plan. It is essential that speakers are able to understand each other and establish effective relationships, making it a fruitful area for linguistic analysis.

There are real benefits to analyzing healthcare talk. Even changing a single word can impact the success of a clinical consultation. Example 6.1 comes from a training video for doctors, used in a pioneering study by Heritage et al. (2007, 2011) in the US and highlighted by Stokoe (2018) in showing valuable applications of close interactional analysis. Consider the question which the doctor asks at lines 4–5:

EXAMPLE 6.1   Training video extract transcribed in Stokoe, 2018: 152, sourced from Heritage et al.'s 2007 study (emphasis added)

```
1 Doctor:   A'right, uh- I understand about th↑: sore throat an' swollen
2           glands.
3               (0.4)
4 Doctor:   Before we deal with that, (0.4) are there ↑any other
5           things: y'd like us to address during this visit,
6 Patient:  No, that's it,
```

DOI: 10.4324/9781003020417-8

Here the doctor asks about 'any other things' the patient might want to address. This question seeks to tackle the issue that patients sometimes lack the opportunity to articulate all their concerns during a consultation – but does it actually work? Heritage et al. (2007) employed Conversation Analysis (CA), an inductive approach for analyzing talk ('talk-in-interaction') in close detail, to find out. Heritage et al. (2007) described how doctors' opening questions, such as, 'What can I do for you today?', normally elicit the expression of a single concern from the patient with additional concerns often not obtained later in the consultation (Heritage et al., 2007). One recommendation for tackling this, provided by communication skills literature, was for the doctor to solicit additional concerns through questions such as, 'Is there anything else we need to take care of today?', just as the doctor does in the excerpt above. Asking a question about 'any other things' seems to make intuitive sense but the response at line 6 is 'No, that's it'. Rather than eliciting additional concerns, asking patients if there is 'anything else' or 'any other things', frequently elicited a 'no' response, even if patients did have other concerns. So, Heritage et al. (2007) found that this recommendation did not work effectively as an interactional strategy.

Part of the explanation Heritage et al. (2007) provide, drawn from findings in earlier research, was that 'any' is negatively polarized when used in questions and invites, or in CA terms tends to 'prefer', a 'no' response more than a 'yes'. The extract they provide from Boyd and Heritage (2006) demonstrates this preference structure in action (Example 6.2):

EXAMPLE 6.2   Extract from Boyd & Heritage, 2006: pp. 169–170 (emphasis added)

```
1    Doctor: ->    An' do you have any other medical problems?
2    Patient:      Uh: no.
3                  (7.0)
4    Doctor:       No heart disease,
5    Patient:      #Hah:.# ((cough))
6    Patient:      No.
7                  (1.3)
8    Doctor: ->    Any lung disease as far as you know:,
9    Patient:      No.
10                 (.)
11   Patient:      Not that I know of.
12                 (.)
13   Doctor: ->    Any diabetes,
14   Patient:      No.
15   Doctor: ->    Have you ever had (uh) surgery?
16                 (0.5)
17   Patient:      I've had four surgeries on my left knee:.
```

Starting with an 'any other medical problems' question at line 1, the doctor sets up some rapid questions about the patient's illness history. The fact that the patient's 'no' answers are prompt and brief seem to confirm that this is the 'preferred' response, with the only non-conforming response at line 17 coming after a lengthy pause of 0.5 seconds and requiring a much longer turn by the patient to elaborate a reason. In this context, where the doctor is quickly running through a history, these 'no' preference questions work well.

However, in the context of asking about additional concerns, Heritage et al. (2007) suggested that this negatively polarized structure for *any*-questions might be a reason patients were not presenting additional concerns. They designed an experiment to test this, substituting the word 'any' with 'some', a positively polarized question, as demonstrated in Example 6.3.

EXAMPLE 6.3   Training video extract transcribed in Stokoe, 2018: 155, sourced from Heritage et al.'s 2007 study (emphasis added)

```
1    Doctor:  A'right.
2             (0.3)
3    Doctor:  I understand about the cough: an' runny nose.=.hh
4             before we deal with that, (.) is there some other issue
5             you'd like us to address, (0.3) during this visit?
6    Patient: Yes w'll I also have this skin thing on my arm,
```

You can see at line 6 that this is modelled as successfully eliciting a patient's concern. They asked groups of doctors to try out the two question formats and the results showed that changing one word had a statistically significant impact on the number of patients reporting additional concerns overall: half of patients in the *any*-question group were left with unmet concerns, compared to only 10% of patients in the *some*-question group.

Heritage et al.'s (2007) study highlights the value in analyzing spoken interaction in these clinical contexts and demonstrates how findings from prior research (such as understanding 'any' as a negatively polarized question) can be applied in exploring issues. It also shows how the tricky question of what makes for an 'effective' healthcare interaction can be at least partly evidenced within talk itself ('endogenously') and not only through retrospective patient satisfaction surveys or other external measures. This chapter will explore avenues and approaches for potential research projects on spoken interaction in healthcare, highlighting frameworks and theories that can be useful to draw on.

6.1.1 In this chapter

The chapter is structured across two broad sections. Section 6.2 addresses practical aspects of designing a research project in this area, including important issues around data access and methods of transcription. Section 6.3 then outlines some key topics in healthcare interactions, presenting studies that approach these using different methods. Section 6.3.1 addresses power asymmetries in 'doctor–patient' interaction and 6.3.2 how culture and identity play out in healthcare encounters in a globalized era. Changes to spoken interaction brought about by technology are a key area of research outlined in 6.3.3 and finally interactions between healthcare teams in 6.3.4. These are important areas you could consider in your own research but are by no means an exhaustive overview of the field.

6.2 Preliminary considerations

Studying verbal interactions in healthcare comes with considerable challenges around access and ethics, as well as unique challenges for handling recorded material. We will outline considerations around deciding a topic and accessing data (6.2.1) and transcribing spoken data (6.2.2).

6.2.1 Deciding on a topic and accessing data

There has been a good deal of research on spoken healthcare encounters, with an extensive body of existing literature. Nevertheless, there are still numerous topics to explore, whatever the scale of your study. You may be able to identify a research gap from reading existing literature, from your own experiences, or from issues raised by patients and healthcare professionals. Even a small-scale study has the opportunity to make an original contribution with applicable findings. Drawing on topics addressed in this chapter, you could consider broad characteristics, such as asymmetric power or cultural identity in healthcare interactions, or you can focus on a single interactional phenomenon, such as how specific types of questions are asked (as with Heritage et al., 2007 above). It is no accident that the chapter started with an example of doctor–patient communication. Doctor–patient relationships are perhaps the most immediately recognizable form of the medical encounter (Gwyn, 2002). Much of the work on spoken interaction in healthcare has focused on these 'dyadic' (between two people), face-to-face consultations between a doctor and a patient. However, it is also important to think beyond this canonical encounter and consider other forms of healthcare interactions. For example, consultations frequently involve additional people, such as interpreters, advocates, and family members, resulting in complex multi-party interactions. Technology is also shifting the modes of healthcare interaction, such as video-mediated and other remote consulting modes (see section 6.3.3). Work between healthcare professionals, such as patient handovers and discussions in multi-disciplinary teams, is also achieved through talk and has started to receive increasing research attention (as in 6.3.4 and Chapter 13).

As outlined in Chapter 3, there are significant practical and ethical challenges to consider in terms of accessing spoken medical interactions. Traditionally, studies of spoken interaction in healthcare have gained data through directly recording patients and healthcare professionals talking. However, this route requires rigorous ethical approvals from your university and sometimes approval from a medical research ethics committee (such as the National Health Service 'Research Ethics Committees' in the UK). Research ethics applications of this kind can be very time consuming and it is worth having a backup option in mind, in case ethical approval is not granted or it simply takes too long. Obtaining this kind of data is therefore most likely to be feasible only in lengthier projects, such as PhD theses and beyond.

There are, however, other routes available for gaining recordings of spoken interaction, and it can be helpful to take a data-driven approach and determine a relevant research question and framework based on the type of data available to you. Firstly, there are pre-existing datasets of medical interactions you can make use of. The spoken component of the original 2007 British National Corpus contains general practice and other medical consultations, recorded in the UK in the 1990s. These are accessible by registering with the University of Lancaster's BNCWeb (http://bncweb.lancs.ac.uk), which provides an interface for searching the corpus. Alternatively, the full corpus of xml files is available for download from the Oxford Text Archive (https://ota.bodleian.ox.ac.uk/repository/xmlui /handle/20.500.12024/2554). Given the size and purpose of the BNC, these medical encounters were transcribed orthographically, rather than using transcription conventions outlined in section 6.3 below, but they do contain valuable detail such as the region of the UK in which the consultation took place. Though the original BNC is now a historic corpus, it provides useful access to a dataset of medical encounters that would otherwise be hard to obtain. In French-speaking contexts there is the CLAPI-FLE corpus (http://clapi.ish-lyon.cnrs.fr), which contains some audio recordings of consultations with dentists and psychologists. A valuable dataset of healthcare interactions in the UK context is also the 'One in a Million' collection of videoed General Practitioner consultations (Barnes, 2017). This resource has purposely been designed to be shared with other researchers, though access requires ethical approval and an application to the research team at the University of Bristol.

For readily accessible data, there are numerous publicly available recordings of spoken communication in healthcare settings, such as television documentaries (e.g. *24 Hours in A&E* and *Hospital* in the UK). These can be useful sources for addressing some types of research questions in short projects, though you will need to keep in mind that this kind of data cannot be treated as 'naturally occurring' due to the design and editing processes involved in such produced content (see ten Have, 2007). It is also possible to look at fictional representations of healthcare interactions, such as in literature or film, perhaps comparing their spoken features to findings on real-life health encounters or looking comparatively at intercultural representations. Just like documentaries, this cannot be treated as 'real', spontaneous interaction, but it is possible to gain insights about patterns in the interactional devices employed to convey meaning in these texts. If fictional representations of healthcare interactions are an area of interest, you should also read Chapter 5 of this book. It is also worth noting that the frameworks outlined in this chapter can be applied to interactions that do not happen face-to-face as in Stommel and Koole's study (2010) in Chapter 8.

A final area to consider is how communication skills are taught to healthcare professionals and assessed, a topic explored in the case study in Chapter 12. Given the importance of spoken interaction in healthcare, communication skills have become a core component of medical education, but often the recommendations do not draw on or match up with evidence from real-life practice. One area might therefore be to look at how findings from health communication research can be effectively applied in training and assessment, such as role-played interactions performed by students, where the same level of ethical approval may not be required to collect data (although do note that you will still need to gain ethical approval from your university and consent any people you record). Despite the complexities of accessing spoken data in healthcare then, there are numerous options to explore and considerable opportunities to produce novel research.

6.3 Transcribing spoken data

Working with recordings of spoken interaction requires preparing your data for analysis, usually through transcription into written form. This enables to you examine an interaction closely and quote extracts in your write-up. Transcription requires making decisions about the level of detail needed. Look again at the excerpts in the Introduction. When we speak, we do not simply use lexical items to convey meaning, but also qualities like intonation (indicated here with an upward arrow, '↑any other'), stress on particular syllables or words (indicated through underlining, '<u>No</u>'), higher or lower volume, speed of delivery and drawn-out sounds, the extended 'e' (indicated here with a colon, 'knee:'), as well as a range of other verbal features, such as fillers ('erm'), noises ('urgh'), and audible breaths. We can overlap with other speakers or interrupt. Even moments where nothing is said, from short micro-pauses during a turn through to longer silences, can be important to how the interaction unfolds and may be useful to represent in your transcript. You will need to think about what sort of detail you will require and how you will transcribe features consistently, according to your research question and the time you have available.

Many researchers typically start by making a standard 'orthographic' transcription of the words that are said, which creates a kind of 'play text' transcript of the talk. This is sufficient for many types of analysis, particularly if you are studying lexical patterns, as corpus approaches do, or if you are looking at broad themes. For more detailed studies, you will need to include other qualities of speech delivery and there are different conventions to draw on here. Conversation Analysis, a method touched on already, has a detailed way of transcribing the features of spoken interaction, referred to as 'Jeffersonian' after Gail Jefferson (for a detailed guide see, Hepburn & Bolden, 2017; Jefferson, 2004). This provides ways of representing the quality of speech delivery, such as intonation, stress, volume and speed, such as those you saw in Examples 6.1, 6.2 and 6.3 above. These conventions are perhaps the most widely used and are recognizable to a broad academic community.

These days you are likely to be working with digital recordings and there are software tools available that can assist with transcription. *Audacity* can help you work with and anonymize your audio. There are also tools that enable you to synchronize your transcripts with the digital recording, creating a 'time stamped' transcript, so that the corresponding moment in the recording can be played. These include tools such as *Transana*, *CLAN*, *ELAN*, and *EXMARaLDA*, detailed further in Hepburn and Golden (2017) with tutorials available online, including Hazel and Mortensen (2015) and Albert (2017).

Transcription decisions can be even more complex when using video data (rather than only audio), since you will need to think about whether features such as gesture, bodily orientation and eye gaze need to be included. CA has methods for representing gaze, gesture and other visible conduct (see Parry, 2010 on dealing with videos in healthcare settings and Chapter 7 of Hepburn & Bolden, 2017 for more general guidance). There are also multimodal methods from Linguistics such as Jewitt (2006) and the MODE approach, demonstrated in section 6.4.3 below.

Whichever transcription convention you decide to follow, make sure you are consistent and provide a key for your reader. You may need to anonymize your transcripts, which involves replacing participants' names with pseudonyms (e.g. replacing the name 'Jen' with 'Liz') or labels ('Participant 1'), as well as removing identifying features such as locations, named institutions, addresses, and telephone numbers (see Chapter 3). Antaki (2002) provides a very useful 'ten guidelines' for anonymizing transcripts. In addition, be aware that there really is no 'neutral' way of transcribing talk and whatever means you choose to represent the recorded interaction will involve transforming your data in some way. For example, CA studies have attempted to represent pronunciation and accent through non-conventional spellings and 'eye dialect' (e.g. 'Howaryuhh' to represent a spoken form of 'How are you?'). Though this can represent pronunciation, there can be an evaluative and potentially political dimension to representing speech this way (Bucholtz, 2000; Roberts, 1997). If accent and pronunciation are the focus of your study, a phonetic transcription system, such as the International Phonetic Alphabet (IPA), might be appropriate for representing short sections of speech.

Overall, while the transcription process can be time consuming, careful transcription becomes part of the analysis and the richness of the data and the understanding you gain make the effort worthwhile. The most important consideration is to choose an approach that is going to help you explore the phenomenon you are interested in. We now turn to the kinds of phenomena that can be investigated.

6.4 Selected studies

6.4.1 Negotiating power and asymmetry in the medical encounter

When a person visits the doctor for a consultation, how much power do they have? Typically, we think of the more powerful speaker as being the health professional – they hold a degree of institutional power and can act as 'gate-keepers' to health advice and treatment. But patients may have some power of negotiation too.

In Chapter 4 you saw Collins et al. (2018) address representations of anti-microbial resistance in news media, a global issue for the use and overuse of antibiotics. This issue also manifests in spoken healthcare encounters, through discussions of when to prescribe antibiotics. Despite numerous health campaigns about the rising risks of antimicrobial resistance in various contexts, inappropriate prescribing continues to be a problem. Looking at paediatric medical contexts in the US, studies by Stivers (2002, 2007) and more recently Stivers and Timmermans (2021) aim to address reasons why this inappropriate prescribing happens. They employ CA to look closely at the talk. Consider Example 6.4 of a mother persuading the doctor to prescribe antibiotics for her child:

EXAMPLE 6.4   Mother negotiating for antibiotic prescription for child, from Stivers (2002)

```
1    DOC:   I think that they probably both have: viral infections
2           'nd .hh (Now) she feels like she's uh little war:m
3           too:, but not too much.

            ((5 lines about fever deleted))

9    DOC:   We::ll I wish I had: better [:: #uh:: [m#
10   MOM:                               [Hhh     [I thought "Oh:
11          ya know maybe-" Cuz ya know usually if it's
12          an ear infection you [give 'em two doses [of=
13   DOC:                        [#Yeah:.#           [Right.
14   MOM:   =antibio[tics and they're [cured.
15   DOC:           [#Y e a h : : .#   [Yeah:.
16   DOC:   No I agree: I mean it's- but it' [s just his ears are=
17   MOM:                                    [Hhhh
18   DOC:   =absolutely perfect =h
19          (0.5)
20   MOM·   Yeah:. I kept sa[ying do your ears hurt?
21   DOC:                   [I mean I could put him o:n an
22          antibiotic and you can see how he is tomorrow that's thuh
23          best- (0.2) ya know- hh
24   MOM:   Alright well- we'll- We'll try it an' I- Tlk
```
[… extract shortened …]

Note how this example, from Stivers' (2002) original study, makes use of the detailed Jeffersonian transcription conventions outlined in 6.3, indicating the length of pauses (e.g. (0.5) at line 19 represents 5 tenths of a second of silence), the stress placed on certain parts if the utterance (e.g. 'absolutely perfect', line 18), the hash sign # to indicate a 'creaky voice' and the colons to indicate a sound has been lengthened (e.g. '[#Y e a h : : .#', line 15). This detail is helpful in looking at the interactional dynamics between the doctor and the patient's mother.

The short extract shows the doctor identifying both the addressee's children as having a viral infection (line 1), which might suggest a prescription of antibiotics was inappropriate. But at lines 12–14 the parent, who has been expressing her desire for antibiotics throughout the consultation, requests this again claiming that it is 'usually' effective, invoking her own medical authority from experience. Although the doctor expresses agreement with her (line 16) he challenges whether there is actually any ear infection to treat: 'but it's just his ears are absolutely perfect' (lines 16–18). However, after a pause the mother continues 'Yeah:. I kept saying do your ears hurt?' and the doctor, quickly coming in in overlap with her turn, addresses the key issue at stake, conceding, 'I mean I could put him o:n an antibiotic' (lines 21–22). The mother immediately accepts with, 'Alright [...] we'll try it' (line 24). This instance indicates how patients can challenge doctors' decisions during the interaction, with the talk becoming a negotiation of authority, rather than the doctor holding a straightforwardly 'powerful' position. Stivers (2002, 2007) and Stivers and Timmermans' (2021) CA studies involved identifying patterns across a large number of consultations, providing convincing findings on the capacity for patients to renegotiate their 'footing' in a medical consultation but also strategies that clinicians can employ to resist this. 'Footing' is a useful term used by Goffman (1981) referring to 'the alignment we take up to ourselves and the others present as expressed in the way we manage the production or reception of an utterance' (128). Participants can shift this alignment in the moment-by-moment interaction, through the cues that they give each other, with moments in the consultation where the asymmetrical relationship can be altered (ten Have, 1991: 146). Micro-analysis of the interaction is therefore a valuable means of explicating this dynamic relationship and the complex social dimensions of decision-making in these encounters.

The doctor–patient relationship and the balance of power in interaction have long been a focus of research, given the expert and institutional setting. The collision of different 'voices', of 'medicine' and the 'lifeworld' (Mishler, 1984) noted earlier, is still important in how we conceptualize communication and may be an area of interest in your own project. The widely advocated model of 'patient-centeredness', which emerged in the 1970s, represented a move away from the authoritarian doctor and the biomedical focus on disease in clinical encounters, towards more personalized care that takes into account patients' concerns and preferences, as well as knowledgeability of their own illness. In this vein, many studies of interaction evidence how patients' ideas, concerns, and expectations can be elicited most effectively in the medical encounter (such as Heritage et al., 2007 in the Introduction) and how doctors and patients can establish a shared decision-making process. Nevertheless, studies such as Roberts and Sarangi (2005), problematize 'patient-centeredness' and some find that asymmetry and the authority of the doctor can also be helpfully oriented to by patients (Pilnick & Dingwall, 2011). You can see the doctor and patient constructively and humorously negotiate professional and institutional authority in the example from Swinglehurst (2014) in section 6.3.3 below. If you are addressing questions of 'power' and 'asymmetry' in your study, you need to approach these carefully, acknowledging that this is a complex phenomenon that might not play out in the way you expect.

6.4.2 Culture and identity in healthcare interactions

We discussed above that healthcare professionals and patients encounter conflicting voices and agendas in medical consultations. This can be more pronounced where speakers' social and cultural identities become relevant in the interaction, an important topic in a globalized era of healthcare. But how can you approach a complex phenomenon like 'identity'? Earlier studies of doctor–patient communication addressed 'identity' as a somewhat pre-given category, such as West (1984) who looked at differences in how male and female doctors talk. However, you have seen already that roles and positions in healthcare encounters are not entirely fixed, but that participants can negotiate their footing during an ongoing interaction. Identity too is 'not simply a reflection of institutional roles and responsibilities but are the results of ongoing interactional negotiations' (Schnurr & Zayts, 2011: 42).

Zayts and Schnurr (2011, 2014) address this in the context of genetic counselling sessions between nurses and clients in Hong Kong, where participants can come from multiple sociocultural and linguistic backgrounds. Genetic counselling is a type of health-professional interaction that involves providing specialist knowledge and support to patients and families to understand the risks, diagnosis, and management of genetic disease. As Zayts and Schnurr (2014) and others (Sarangi, 2000) have noted, this counselling is a complex activity, with differing expectations of the purpose, aims, and practices of those participating.

Zayts and Schnurr (2014) draw on Interactional Sociolinguistics to address the discursive construction of the nurses' identities. Interactional Sociolinguistics combines the interest in the micro-analysis of spoken interaction we noted above with a more macro understanding of the context in which the interactions take place (Gumperz, 1999). Unlike CA then, interactional sociolinguistics looks beyond the talk itself to also consider the 'communicative ecology' and wider sociocultural context in which speakers interact (Auer & Roberts, 2011), often addressing aspects such as intercultural misunderstandings and the different backgrounds and interactional resources speakers have. It has become a widely used approach for researching healthcare interactions because of its ability to take into account social relationships between participants in the institutional context of healthcare (e.g. Sarangi & Roberts, 1999). In conducting their study, Zayts and Schnurr used recordings of 150 genetic counselling sessions to look closely at interactions, but also used interviews and questionnaires to gather ethnographic information (see 6.3.3 below on ethnography) and drew on patients' own understandings of the consultations (Zayts & Schnurr, 2014: 350–1). In theorizing identity, they draw on Bucholtz and Hall (2005), particularly the idea of the 'relationality principle', where '[i]dentities are intersubjectively constructed through several, often overlapping, complementary relations' (Bucholtz & Hall, 2005: 598). This is a seminal sociolinguistic approach to identity also referred to in Chapter 8.

Have a look at the following Example 6.5 from Zayts and Schnurr's dataset, a telephone consultation with a Filipina mother whose newborn baby has been diagnosed with a genetic disorder (G6PD deficiency), a condition she has not heard of before:

EXAMPLE 6.5 Telephone genetic counselling session with a Filipina
mother, from Zayts and Schnurr (2014: 361–2) N – Nurse,
M – Mother

1. N: Okay? So, firstly, you don't give any medicine to your baby
2.   by your own.
3. M: Okay.
4. N: .h actually are you Indian or Pakistan?
5. M: No, eh is eh Filipino.
6. N: Oh! Filipino. So do you have any (.) I mean traditional herb,
7.   (.) or medicine in Philippine for the baby?
8. M: No.
9. N: No, so that's fine. So you just .h ah stick to the rules, okay?
10.   No matter it is your family ah traditional medicine or
11.   whatever. Just don't give the baby any kind of medicine or
12.   drug without seeing doctor.
        [10 turns omitted]
13.   Don't feed your baby with the broad bean, (.) or the fava bean.
14.   Do you see the number three?
15.   ((refers to patient information leaflet))
16. M: (2.0) Um: where?
17. N: Number three. [Do you see?]
18. M: [Number three?]
19. N: Yea, the broad bean. So (.) ah only the broad bean (.)
20.   the baby cannot eat. Okay?
21. M: Okay.
22. N: Okay? All other kind of food, (.) he can eat.
23. M: What does it mean of broad bean?
24. N: Broad bean, it is a kind of bean.
25. M: Bean?
26. N: Yeah, look like the kidney shape. And it is quite big. .h
27.   And some people use it as a snack. .h So if you go to
28.   those shops selling the snack, you ask them for the broad
29.   bean, they would show you. Usually they are very (.)
30.   quite big, I mean compare with other kind of bean. Okay?
31. M: Okay.
32. N: They are quite big and slightly brownish color.
33. M: Okay.
34. N: And some are (.) have the brown hard coat, okay? And look
35.   like a kidney. You- you- you know how the kidney look like?
36. M: (.) Sorry?
37. N: Kidney.
38. M: Kidney bean?
39. N: Yeah, it look like the kidney, the shape.
40. M: Oh, yeah.

Note that this is a different type of transcript to the conversation analytic conventions you saw in the previous section, with some similar notation showing pauses '(.)' and overlaps in square brackets, but with the punctuation, such as question marks and full stops, largely following standard orthographic conventions. This is perhaps a more simplified transcript, but it is sufficient for examining the discursive negotiation of identity that Zayts and Schnurr (2014) focus on. If you are transcribing talk for your study, you will need to make similar decisions about the level of detail required.

In this example, Zayts and Schnurr describe how the nurse adopts a role of 'cultural-broker', mediating and explicating culturally specific ideas, such as the 'traditional herbs or medicine' she asks about at lines 6–7, that might be given to babies in the mother's home country. This is 'important in this context as there are certain Chinese medicinal products and other substances which individuals with the condition should not be exposed to' (2014: 362). She then moves on to describe foods the baby must not have; 'broad beans' at line 13. There is some confusion over the understanding of 'broad bean' (line 23 and 25), which is tricky to manage in this remote telephone consultation. The nurse describes its shape (line 26) but also explains how some people in Hong Kong eat it as a snack (line 27). In doing so Zayts and Schnurr suggest that:

> The nurse thus moves beyond a description of the bean's appearance and sets up two different, and in this case opposing, subject positions for the mother ('you') on the one hand, and local Hong Kong people ('they') on the other hand. Interestingly, the nurse positions herself in between these two poles: she is not claiming an in-group status with either the mother or the Hong Kong locals. Thus, the mother is constructed as a foreigner who is provided with crucial information by the nurse who is at the same time portrayed as a mediator and facilitator between the (foreign) client and the locals.
>
> (*Zayts & Schnurr, 2014: 364*)

Here then, the nurse is taking on the role of knowledgeable cultural mediator, spelling out specific cultural practices and responding to the demands of a diverse context like Hong Kong. The client is positioned against this as 'less knowledgeable' and perhaps 'non-local'. Across the data, Zayts and Schnurr identify the range of roles that nurses draw on and sometimes reject during these interactions. This includes invoking a role as a medical expert and a professional giving advice, but also the role of counsellor in responding to the client's psychological concerns, co-decision maker, as well as the 'cultural-broker' role shown above. In doing so, nurses negotiate and manage 'the sometimes competing expectations and agendas of their institutions and profession, their clients, and themselves' (Schnurr & Zayts, 2011: 364). Analyzing roles and identity construction can be a useful way of understanding the interactional complexities of clinical encounters and the many roles that healthcare provider and patient negotiate.

Intercultural understanding and identities within the interaction are important areas for research on spoken healthcare communication, as healthcare professionals and patient populations become more diverse. The contemporary relevance of this is highlighted by Cox et al. (2021) in their call for interdisciplinary research on communication with migrant patients in emergency settings during the Covid-19 crisis. Cox and Maryns (2021) use linguistic ethnographic methods (an approach outlined in the next section) to highlight some of the cultural and linguistic miscommunication that can arise in emergency departments. There is wide scope then for linguists to conduct further research in the area of culture and identity.

6.4.3 Incorporating technology into health interactions

Technological changes have impacts throughout healthcare, including on how we interact. Chapters 7 and 8 address this in written contexts. In spoken contexts, interactions with technology present benefits and challenges. The GP and scholar Deborah Swinglehurst became interested in how the technology of the 'electronic patient record' (EPR) took a central role in day-to-day interactions in primary care consultations (Swinglehurst, 2014, 2015). The EPR became the main form of medical record keeping for UK patients and is usually visible on a computer screen during a consultation for a practitioner to refer to. Importantly it is also used for medical auditing through the 'Quality Outcomes Framework' (QOF), which makes up a large proportion of a GP surgery's remuneration. Recognizing the EPR as a complex phenomenon, Swinglehurst took a 'linguistic ethnographic' approach. Linguistic Ethnography draws on a range of methods, including close analysis of spoken data, but also incorporating a deep understanding of the context of a communicative event, often including participants' own perspectives on their practices. This involves the researcher conducting fieldwork (see also 3.3.4 in this book) and interacting with participants to gain understanding of the context (for a detailed introduction, see Copland & Creese, 2015; Snell et al., 2015, and also Chapter 8, section 8.3.3 on digital ethnography). In this study, Swinglehurst conducted recordings and interactional analysis of clinical encounters, but incorporated her own understanding as a GP of institutional structures and her observations of routines within GP practices, which she recorded through ethnographic fieldnotes.

The recordings of the consultations required careful decisions about how to transcribe complex, multimodal actions in GP consultations. Swinglehurst started by conducting repeat viewings of videos to decide what level of detail was required (2015: p. 101). She employed Jeffersonian transcription conventions for the verbal talk, but adapted a multimodal transcription system from Jewitt (2006) to represent bodily conduct and the information displayed on the EPR in adjacent columns. You can learn more about this transcription approach through the MODE online resource (https://mode.ioe.ac.uk). An example transcript from Swinglehurst (2014) is given in Example 6.6.

EXAMPLE 6.6   Data extract 'My computer's asked me … ', from Swinglehurst (2014)

Time	D P	Words spoken /sounds	Bodily conduct	EPR Screen
14.32	D	now my computer's	D - > EPR. D points to screen	Medications screen.
		asked me whether you smoke	D - > EPR, L hand to mouth; P --> EPR;	QOF alert showing in bottom R corner: QOF Recent Smoking Data (displays throughout consultation)
		(1.2)	D - > P; P - > EPR	
14.35	P	uhm	P - > EPR	
		(1.0)		
14.36	P	yes (.) no	P - > EPR; D - > P	
		(1.0)	P - > D	
14.38	D	he what's [that mean	D - > EPR, laughing	
	P	[I've had one in the last three days	D < -> P	
14.41	D	right (.) so (.) very occasionally	D < -> P	
14.43	P	yeah (0.2) I'm (.) I'm very much a s:ocial smoker nowadays=		
14.46	D	= so with- in a (0.2) in a week uhm how many do you get through °d'you think°		
14.49	P	well last week I think I had three		
14.52	D	right (0.4) right		
		(5.0)	D turns - > EPR; P - > D. At 14.57 D turns to P again	
Transcript not shown – doctor establishes that patient smoked three cigarettes last week and suggests it would be better for patient's general health if she could "ignore them", since although it is not doing "horrendous damage" it is still keeping the "receptors flapping"				
15.29	D	so (0.2) y'know obviously	D - > EPR; P - > D	
		°<as your doctor > I have to advise you that you shouldn't°	D < -> P; D using highly stylised voice	
		(1.6)	D nods, smiling	

In this extract, the doctor has finished addressing the patient's gynaecological problem and moves on to address an institutional requirement, responding to an EPR prompt displayed in the bottom right of her computer screen – a 'QOF alert' to ask about smoking. Here, at 14.32, the doctor re-orients to look at the screen, pointing to it as she announces 'now my computer's asked me whether you smoke'. The patient then also looks towards the EPR and hesitates in her response (14.35–14.36). Swinglehurst suggests that,

> [h]ere, the doctor attributes agency for her opening utterance to the EPR, suggesting that the EPR is the author of her words (Goffman, 1981). This is effective in introducing some attributional distance between herself and the delicate question she asks of the patient (Clayman, 1992) whilst also identifying her professional authority as somehow at issue.
>
> *(Swinglehurst, 2015: 103)*

A little later, at 15:29, there is an interesting moment in which the doctor explicitly shifts the 'footing' for the participants, claiming the professional authority '<as your doctor>' when advising the patient not to smoke. This invokes her professional 'identity' to legitimize her advice but also orienting humorously to an institutional requirement to perform this action, following the QOF question and gaining a smile from the patient. The example illustrates Swinglehurst's findings about how clinicians must make 'on the spot' judgements in how to incorporate the institutional voice of the EPR into their interactions and demonstrates a type of 'hybrid discourse' (Roberts & Sarangi, 1999), combining both 'professional' and 'institutional' identities. These are valuable strategies for managing relationships with patients when the voice of the medical institution 'intrudes' upon the discussion.

Swinglehurst's approach shows the ways in which complex interactions with technology can be approached. For Swinglehurst, the ability to deal with the complexity of social life was one of the appeals of Linguistic Ethnography, addressing the interface between the details of interaction but also broader institutional practices in which it is situated. Linking these dimensions can be challenging, as Swinglehurst (2015) highlights, particularly as it involves managing the collection and analysis of many different types of data. But there are fascinating insights to be had in combining some of detailed micro-analytic insights we have discussed for CA with broader understandings of the social and institutional context.

Technologically driven changes to healthcare encounters were particularly apparent during the Covid-19 pandemic, during which remote methods of consulting became widely used. An interesting conversation analytic study of the challenges of video consultations was conducted by a team at the University of Oxford (Greenhalgh et al., 2020; Shaw et al., 2020), looking at difficulties encountered and providing practical, research-evidenced advice. For example, to look at issues caused by 'latency' over video consultations, i.e when there is a delay in the transmission of talk, they made a 'dual' Jeffersonian transcript of what the two different parties actually hear, side-by-side, given in Example 6.7 below. This is a consultation about heart failure in which the patient is talking to a specialist nurse.

EXAMPLE 6.7   Latency disrupting conversational flow in a video
consultation for heart failure. (Ns: nurse; Pt: patient),
from Shaw et al. (2020: 12) (CC BY 4.0)

What the patient heard (ie, recorded at the patient's end)	What the nurse heard (ie, recorded at the nurse's end)
| ```
01 Pt: uhm I told you about playing
02     croquet? as you know I
03     played croquet last year;
04     h[hh this year .h I'm
05 Ns: [yeah,
06 Pt: struggling to complete
07     one round.
08     (0.5)
09     without having to sit d[own
10 Ns:                        [are
11     you really;
12 Pt: yeah.
13     (0.5)
14     u:hm I'm gonna keep on at
15     it, I'[ve got a-]
16 Ns:      [and is  i]t a pos-
17     (1.0)
18 Pt: sorry,
19     (1.5)
20     .hh[h
21 Ns:    [yeah go on¿
22 Pt: I've g[ot-      ]
23 Ns:       [y'r gonna ]keep
24     on,
25     (0.4)
26 Pt: yeah I've got a .hh
27     competition at ((place
28     name)) tomorrow
``` | ```
Pt: uhm I told you about playing
    croquet? as you know I
    [played croquet last year;
Ns: [yeah,
Pt: .hhh this year I'm
    struggling to complete
    one round.
Ns: are you really;
Pt: without having to sit down.
    (0.6)
Pt: [yeah.
Ns: [(hm)
    (0.4)
    and is i[t   a    p o s-]
Pt:        [I'm gonna kee]p
    on at it, I've-
    (1.9)
Pt: sorry,
Ns: g- yeah go on¿
    (0.5)
Ns: y'r gonna keep on,
    (0.2)
Pt: I've dot- (1.0) yeah I've got
    a .hh competition at ((place
    name)) tomorrow.
``` |

Latency is common in video-interactions when the connection drops and can be seen in the extracts here, where the speakers hear different things, making the interaction challenging. As the patient tells the nurse about his back problem, the nurse seems to interrupt (line 16). This 'interruption' is not deliberate on the part of the nurse but a result of the lag – she just hadn't realized the patient had begun talking again because of the delay. The result is overlapping talk and some confusion. Eventually, both speakers stop, and it takes a series of silences and repair sequences (such as the patient's 'sorry' (line 18), and the nurse's 'yeah go on' (line 21)) before the patient can resume his account that 'I've got a competition tomorrow' (line 26–27).

Face-to-face or 'co-present' conversation has relatively ordered turn-taking and we find swapping turns quite easy, often minimizing silence and overlaps. Shaw et al. (2020) found that latency is much more tolerated in remote consultations, or at least, up to a point – about 0.2 of a second to be specific. This might be a relatively long silence in face-to-face consultations but is less significant when talking remotely. However, longer lags (about half-second gaps and above) really seemed to interfere with the turn-taking, resulting in silences, overlapping talk or interruptions, as with the example above. Sometimes these problems were resolved quickly and in other cases they took longer to fix. In most cases in Shaw et al.'s (2020) data, where latency caused disruptions like this, participants relied on the same strategies that might be used in face-to-face conversation to try and get things back on track, such as requesting repair ('sorry?') or repeating the last thing they heard, and these strategies generally worked. Nevertheless, these repair issues happen more frequently in remote consulting, with 'safety-netting' therefore required by the healthcare professional to check there have not been misunderstandings during the consultation. There is much to understand about how technology impacts upon our healthcare interactions, both in institutional settings and outside.

6.4.4 Relationships in healthcare teams

So far, we have largely looked at interactions between healthcare professionals and 'lay persons', such as patients or families. This has been an important focus for health communication research, where the 'voice of medicine' and the 'voice of the lifeworld' meet. However, other types of spoken communication are also important, such as communication between healthcare professionals.

Atkins and Chalupnik (2021) and Chalupnik and Atkins (2020) look into what makes for effective interactions between medics training in emergency medical teams. They focus on communication skills training for team leaders, analyzing simulated scenarios that junior doctors perform and are assessed on. Although these are simulated scenarios, which do not hold the same pressures as real trauma incidents (see Chapter 12 on simulations), these assessed interactions were nevertheless acutely time-sensitive and give some insight into the types of communication skills required for entry into the medical profession. Have a look at Example 6.8, which is a simulated scenario meant to provide doctors with practice in leading medical teams. The doctor being assessed here, Colin (DOC), is an experienced junior doctor in the hospital's Emergency Department. In his team are Linda (NRS), a nurse, and Gareth (F2D), a more junior doctor, who are themselves emergency care professionals. In this opening clip, Linda has informed Colin about a patient who is soon to arrive in the Emergency Department:

EXAMPLE 6.8   Emergency medical team interaction, from Atkins and
Chalupnik (2021) (emphasis added)

```
36 DOC: What we'll do (.) in the meantime,
37 F2D: Yeah
38 DOC: Before the trauma team arrive (.) I'll do the initial survey,
39 F2D: Yeah,
40 DOC: But if I can get you to pla:n (0.2) um (.) and get some I V access.
41      [>In case] we need it< um (.) when he [comes  in  so] F P C (.) coag,
42 F2D: [Yeah:    ]                           [Yeah (.) sure]
43 F2D: Yep.
44        (0.4)
45 DOC: Blood for a cross match sam[ple.]
46 F2D:                           [Yep.]
47        (0.2)
48 DOC: And routine biochemistry and the venous blood gas:
49 F2D: Okay yeah I can do that yeh.
50 DOC: I V access (.) large (xxx) please.
51 F2D: Yep
52 DOC: Would you mind (.) doing initial circuit observations.
53 NRS: [Yeah]
54 DOC: [Sats blood pressure cu[ff, ]
55 NRS:                       [Yeah]
56 DOC: E C G monitoring=
57 NRS:                  =Yeah I can do that.
   [...]
67 DOC: Can we get erm a ↑bear hugger- a warmer ↑underneath¿
68 NRS: On the ↑troll[ey ye:p,         ]
69 DOC:             [>if that's alright<]
70        (1.6)
71 DOC: Fantastic.
72 NRS: Here it is.
```

This doctor performs well in the assessed simulation, completing all the tasks
within the allotted time and gaining high scores from the examiner. Atkins and
Chalupnik (2021) were particularly interested in how requests were performed
by the team leader, some of which are highlighted in bold the example. Even this
short excerpt shows that he used a good deal of 'indirectness' and 'polite' forms
in his talk, such as 'Would you mind … ' (52), 'Can we get … ' (67) using the
collective 'we' for the team even though this request is being directed to a specific team member. These delegated tasks are accepted quickly by the recipients
('Okay yeah I can do that yeh'. l. 49).

Atkins and Chalupnik approached this using frameworks from the field of
Pragmatics. As outlined in Chapter 2, Pragmatics is a very broad area but can
be defined as an approach to language and meaning that places *context* at the
centre of analysis, with speakers drawing on their knowledge, surroundings
and social relationships to make sense of what is said. For example, it is fairly
straightforward for the team member in the scenario above to understand that
the collective 'we' in 'Can we get … ', rather than requesting an action of the
whole team, actually means a specific task has been allocated to him. Pragmatics
encompasses areas such as 'speech acts' (how actions are achieved through talk
(Austin, 1962, Searle, 1976)), and theories about how our interactional choices
are guided by the maintenance of interpersonal relationships, such as 'politeness'
(Brown & Levinson, 1987) or 'rapport management' (Spencer-Oatey, 2000).
It addresses how we understand 'indirectness' in interaction, such as the ways
we convey a message through hints and implied meanings, often as a way to

be polite and maintain social relationships (Searle, 1975, see Haugh, 2014 for a recent study of the relationship between politeness and implicature). Pragmatic theories of politeness and indirectness are a valuable means of analyzing interaction and you will see them employed again in Chapter 7 in looking at aspects such the pragmatic function of expressions of empathy and mitigating potential 'face threat' in online advice-giving (see Chapters 1 and 2 on the notion of 'face').

Overall, the requests that Atkins and Chalupnik (2021) address show that the trainees who used more indirect and mitigated forms in their delegation of tasks were evaluated positively for leadership skills. Furthermore, these team leaders achieved tasks more quickly. This observation challenges claims in both the pragmatics and health communication literature about directness being necessary in emergency situations, where 'politeness norms' can be suspended. Bezemer et al. (2016) identified similar patterns in surgical team interactions using linguistic ethnography and some of the MODE methods for multimodal analysis of video data outlined in section 6.3.3. As you can see, medical team interactions provide valuable opportunities for research, approachable using a number of the methods outlined in this chapter.

6.5 Concluding remarks

Spoken communication is an important area for research in healthcare. Close analysis, using transcripts of recorded talk, enables us to see the detail of where things can go wrong, as well as best practice for healthcare communication, helping to answer questions about how to talk effectively with patients or with medical professionals. As an ever-evolving context, important new research questions emerge all the time, such as those around power, identity, interactions with technology, and between medical teams that we have addressed in this chapter. Although spoken data can be hard to access in healthcare, we have highlighted potential routes available for studies at various scales, along with some of the practicalities around transcription and methods. Though challenging, research in this area has potential for beneficial applications, making a project in this area enormously rewarding.

Further readings

Brookes, G., & Hunt, D. (Eds.). (2021). *Analysing health communication: Discourse approaches.* Springer Nature (See Chapter 2 on conversation analysis, Chapter 3 on interactional sociolinguistics and Chapter 11 on pragmatics).

Harvey, K., & Koteyko, N. (2013). *Exploring health communication: Language in action* (Routledge introductions to applied linguistics). Routledge. (See Part I on Spoken health communication, pp. 5–38).

Heritage, J., & Maynard, D. W. (Eds.). (2006). *Communication in medical care: Interaction between primary care physicians and patients.* Cambridge University Press.

References

Albert, S. (2017). *Digital transcription for EM/CA research* [Website]. Retrieved October 23, 2022, from https://saulalbert.net/digital-transcription/

Antaki, C. (2002). An introductory tutorial in conversation analysis. Retrieved from http://ca-tutorials.lboro.ac.uk/sitemenu.htm

Atkins, S., & Chalupnik, M. (2021). Pragmatics: Leadership and team communication in emergency medicine training. In G. Brookes & D. Hunt (Eds.), *Analysing health communication: Discourse approaches* (pp. 271–299). Palgrave Macmillan.

Auer, P., & Roberts, C. (2011). Introduction: John Gumperz and the indexicality of language. *Text & Talk – An Interdisciplinary Journal of Language, Discourse & Communication Studies*, *31*(4), 381–393.

Austin, J. L. (1962). *How to do things with words*. Clarendon.

Barnes, R. (2017). *One in a million: A study of primary care consultations* [dataset]. https://doi.org/10.5523/bris.l3sq4s0w66ln1x20sye7s47wv

Bezemer, J., Murtagh, G., Cope, A., & Kneebone, R. (2016). Surgical decision making in a teaching hospital: A linguistic analysis. *ANZ Journal of Surgery*, *86*(10), 751–755.

Boyd, E., & Heritage, J. (2006). Taking the history: Questioning during comprehensive history taking. In J. Heritage & D. W. Maynard (Eds.), *Communication in medical care: Interaction between primary care physicians and patients* (pp. 151–184). Cambridge University Press.

Brown, P., & Levinson, S. C. (1987). *Politeness: Some universals in language usage*. Cambridge University Press.

Bucholtz, M. (2000). The politics of transcription. *Journal of Pragmatics*, *32*(10), 1439–1465.

Bucholtz, M., & Hall, K. (2005). Identity and interaction: A sociocultural linguistic approach. *Discourse Studies*, *7*(4–5), 585–614.

Chałupnik, M., & Atkins, S. (2020). "Everyone happy with what their role is?": A pragmalinguistic evaluation of leadership practices in emergency medicine training. *Journal of Pragmatics*, *160*, 80–96.

Clayman, S. E. (1992). Footing in the achievement of neutrality: The case of news-interview discourse. In P. Drew & J. Heritage (Eds.), *Talk at work: Interaction in institutional settings* (pp. 163–198). Cambridge University Press.

Collins, L. C., Jaspal, R., & Nerlich, B. (2018). Who or what has agency in the discussion of antimicrobial resistance in UK news media (2010–2015)? A transitivity analysis. *Health*, *22*(6), 521–540.

Copland, F., & Creese, A. (2015). *Linguistic ethnography: Collecting, analysing and presenting data*. Sage.

Cox, A., Iedema, R., Li, S., Sabbe, M., Salaets, H., & Dauby, N. (2021). Adding barriers to barriers during the COVID-19 pandemic: A call for interdisciplinary research on communication with migrant patients in the emergency department. *European Journal of Emergency Medicine*, *28*(1), 5–6. Retrieved from https://journals.lww.com/euro-emergencymed/Fulltext/2021/01000/Adding_barriers_to_barriers_during_the_COVID_19.3.aspx

Cox, A., & Maryns, K. (2021). Multilingual consultations in urgent medical care. *The Translator*, *27*(1), 75–93. https://doi.org/10.1080/13556509.2020.1857501

Goffman, E. (1981). *Forms of talk*. University of Pennsylnvania Press.

Greenhalgh, T., Wherton, J., Shaw, S., & Morrison, C. (2020). Video consultations for Covid-19. *BMJ*, *368*, m998.

Gumperz, J. (1999). On interactional sociolinguistic method. In S. Sarangi & C. Roberts (Eds.), *Talk, work, and institutional order: Discourse in medical, mediation, and management settings* (pp. 453–471). Mouton de Gruyter.

Gwyn, R. (2002). *Communicating health and illness*. Sage.

Haugh, M. (2014). *Im/Politeness implicatures*. De Gruyter Mouton. https://doi.org/10.1515/9783110240078

Hazel, S., & Mortensen, J. (2015). CLAN Manual – For workshop training. LangSoc Lab, Roskilde University. Retrieved from http://spencerhazel.net/wp-content/uploads/2015/09/CLAN-manual-LangSoc-Lab.pdf

Hepburn, A., & Bolden, G. B. (2017). *Transcribing for social research*. Sage.

Heritage, J., & Robinson, J. D. (2011). 'Some' versus 'any' medical issues: Encouraging patients to reveal their unmet concerns. In C. Antaki (Ed.), *Applied conversation analysis* (pp. 15–31). Palgrave Macmillan.

Heritage, J., Robinson, J. D., Elliott, M. N., Beckett, M., & Wilkes, M. (2007). Reducing patients' unmet concerns in primary care: The difference one word can make. *Journal of General Internal Medicine, 22*(10), 1429–1433.

Jefferson, G. (2004). Glossary of transcript symbols with an introduction. In G. H. Lerner (Ed.), *Conversation analysis: Studies from the first generation* (pp. 13–34). John Benjamins.

Jewitt, C. (2006). *Technology, literacy and learning: A multimodal approach*. Routledge.

Mishler, E. (1984). *The discourse of medicine: Dialectics of medical interviews*. Greenwood Publishing Group.

Parry, R. (2010). Video-based conversation analysis. In I. Bourgeault, R. Dingwall, R. de Vries (Eds.), *Sage handbook of qualitative methods in health research* (pp. 373–396). Sage.

Pilnick, A., & Dingwall, R. (2011). On the remarkable persistence of asymmetry in doctor/patient interaction: A critical review. *Social Science and Medicine, 72*(8), 1374–1382.

Roberts, C. (1997). Transcribing talk: Issues of representation. *TESOL Quarterly, 31*(1), 167–172.

Roberts, C., & Sarangi, S. (1999). Hybridity in gatekeeping discourse: Issues of practical relevance for the researcher. In S. Sarangi & C. Roberts (Eds.), *Talk, work and institutional order* (pp. 473–503). Mouton de Gruyter.

Roberts, C., & Sarangi, S. (2005). Theme-oriented discourse analysis of medical encounters. *Medical Education, 39*(6), 632–640.

Sarangi, S. (2000). Activity types, discourse types and interactional hybridity: The case of genetic counseling. In M. Coulthard & S. Sarangi (Eds.), *Discourse and social life* (pp. 1–27). Longman.

Schnurr, S., & Zayts, O. (2011). Constructing and contesting leaders. An analysis of identity construction at work. In J. Angouri & M. Marra (Eds.), *Constructing identities at work* (pp. 40–60). Palgrave.

Searle, J. (1975). Indirect speech acts. In P. Cole & J. Morgan (Eds.), *Syntax and semantics, vol. 3: Speech acts* (pp. 59–82). Academic Press.

Searle, J. R. (1976). A classification of illocutionary acts. *Language in Society, 5*(1), 1–23.

Shaw, S. E., Seuren, L. M., Wherton, J., Cameron, D., Vijayaraghavan, S., Morris, J., Bhattacharya, S., & Greenhalgh, T. (2020). Video consultations between patients and clinicians in diabetes, cancer, and heart failure services: Linguistic ethnographic study of video-mediated interaction. *Journal of Medical Internet Research, 22*(5), e18378.

Snell, J., Shaw, S., & Copland, F. (Eds.). (2015). *Linguistic ethnography* (pp. 14–50). Palgrave Macmillan.

Spencer-Oatey, H. (Eds.). (2000). *Culturally speaking. Managing rapport through talk across cultures*. Continuum.

Stivers, T. (2002). Participating in decisions about treatment: Overt parent pressure for antibiotic medication in pediatric encounters. *Social Science and Medicine, 54*(7), 1111–1130.

Stivers, T. (2007). *Prescribing under pressure: Parent-physician conversations and antibiotics.* Oxford University Press.

Stivers, T., & Timmermans, S. (2021). Arriving at no: Patient pressure to prescribe antibiotics and physicians' responses. *Social Science and Medicine, 290*, 114007.

Stokoe, E. (2018). *Talk: The science of conversation.* Hachette UK.

Stommel, W., & Koole, T. (2010). The online support group as a community: A micro-analysis of the interaction with a new member. *Discourse Studies, 12*(3), 357–378.

Swinglehurst, D. (2014). Displays of authority in the clinical consultation: A linguistic ethnographic study of the electronic patient record. *Social Science and Medicine, 118*, 17–26.

Swinglehurst, D. (2015). How linguistic ethnography may enhance our understanding of electronic patient records in health care settings. In J. Snell, S. Shaw & F. Copland (Eds.), *Linguistic ethnography* (pp. 90–109). Palgrave Macmillan.

ten Have, P. (1991). Talk and institution: A reconsideration of the 'asymmetry' of doctor-patient interaction. In D. Boden & D. H. Zimmerman (eds.) *Talk and social structure: Studies in ethnomethodology and conversation analysis* (pp. 138–163). Polity Press.

ten Have, P. (2007). *Doing conversation analysis.* Sage Publications.

West, C. (1984). When the doctor is a "lady": Power, status and gender in physician-patient encounters. *Symbolic Interaction, 7*(1), 87–106.

Zayts, O., & Schnurr, S. (2011). Laughter as medical providers' resource: Negotiating informed choice in prenatal genetic counseling. *Research on Language and Social Interaction, 44*(1), 1–20.

Zayts, O., & Schnurr, S. (2014). More than 'information provider' and 'counselor': Constructing and negotiating roles and identities of nurses in genetic counseling sessions. *Journal of Sociolinguistics, 18*(3), 345–369.

7
DIGITAL TECHNOLOGIES AND HEALTH TALK ONLINE

7.1 Introduction

Dr Liz O'Riordan, a breast cancer surgeon who was diagnosed with breast cancer at the age of 40, makes the following comment in a 2018 news article about her experience of becoming a patient:

> I used to tell all my patients not to Google breast cancer. I naively thought I could give them all the information they needed.
>   But it's the first thing I did when I got my biopsy result, and I'm an expert.

> *(O'Riordan, 2010)*

If even a specialist turns to an online search engine after a diagnosis, it is not surprising that study after study has found that the vast majority of internet users do the same when they are concerned about a health condition (e.g. Wang et al.'s 2021 review of research on health-information-seeking practices from around the world).

As you may know from first-hand experience, there is a wide variety of websites that one can land on when searching for health-related information, from official sites run by national health providers to blogs by people who choose to share their personal stories of illness online. Figure 7.1 provides some examples.

In this chapter, we show how linguistic analysis can contribute to a better understanding of interactions between online experts and patients, and of the ways in which patients and the general public respond to health news and healthcare services online.

DOI: 10.4324/9781003020417-9

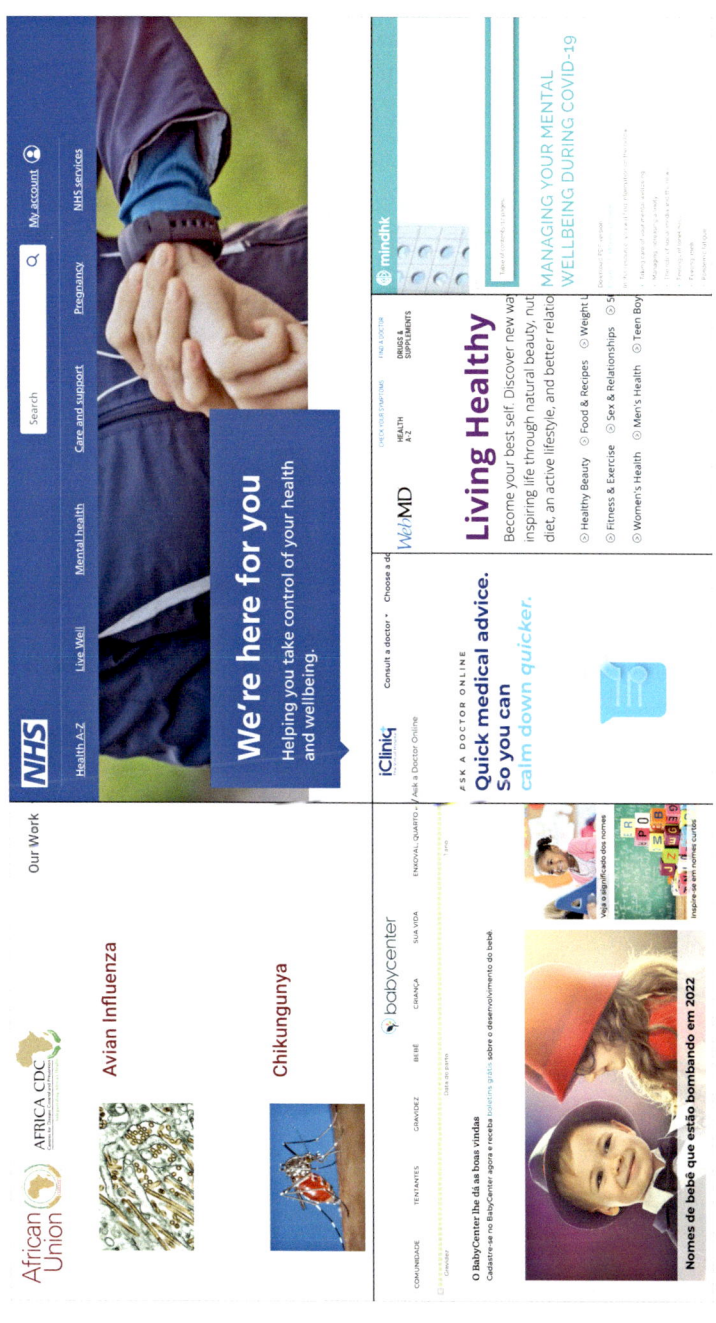

FIGURE 7.1   Collage of health–related websites

Zhang (2021), for example, points out the use of first-person *plural* pronoun in this (translated) extract from a doctor's response to a pregnant advice-seeker on a Chinese medical website:

EXAMPLE 7.1

> You can consult me at any time and over the long term; that way, *we* can give the baby a timely, comprehensive, and proper answer! *Our* common goal is for the baby to grow up healthy and strong.
>
> *(Zhang, 2021: 821; emphasis added)*

Zhang suggests that the use of 'we' to include both doctor and patient establishes an empathic relationship in a context where the two people do not know each other, and also makes it more likely that the patient will leave positive feedback on this particular doctor's performance and return for further advice in the future.

7.1.1 In this chapter

In the rest of this chapter, we begin with linguistic approaches to advice-seeking, advice-giving, and empathy on websites where professionals respond to health concerns from members of the general public, including particularly teenagers and young people. We then discuss studies of comments on online news articles about health-related topics and online feedback on health. As online data is potentially available in large quantities, the studies we consider in the course of the chapter tend to combine quantitative and qualitative approaches to sizeable datasets, often by making use of corpus linguistic techniques. In the next chapter, we show how these and other analytical tools are relevant to the analysis of peer-to-peer interactions about, or lived-experience descriptions of illness online, for example on a forum dedicated to people with cancer and their families.

7.2 Preliminary considerations

The considerations we mentioned in previous chapters with regard to selecting a topic apply to this chapter too. Here we will consider issues that apply specifically to the selection and analysis of data from online sources, and that are therefore relevant to the current chapter and the next one.

7.2.1 Selecting sources of data

The rationale for selecting an online source of data tends to involve a combination of considerations of relevance, ethical issues, and ease of access.

With regard to relevance, studies of online interactions about health usually emphasize the importance of the selected websites or webpages. For example, three of the studies we discuss in this chapter are concerned with online sources of advice for teenagers and young adults (Locher, 2006, Harvey, 2012, Mullany et al., 2015). All three studies make a case for providing young people with the opportunity to ask for health advice anonymously, especially with regard to sensitive and/or embarrassing concerns, and highlight the insights that can be gained into young people's lived experience by analyzing their requests for advice.

Most studies in this area also provide some evidence of the popularity of the relevant website as part of the justification for selecting a particular source of online health advice (cf. our comments in Chapter 5 on selecting published narratives analysis based on best-seller lists). For example, Zhang (2021) justifies the selection of the medical consultation website 'Chunyu Doctor' by citing independent evidence that it is among the top five online healthcare platforms in China. Locher (2010: 47) provides more specific quantitative support for selecting a particular University's online health advice service, by pointing out that, at the time of data collection, it received 2,000 requests for advice from students per week. Collins (2019) combines qualitative and quantitative considerations for analyzing readers' online comments on two health-related news reports. On the one hand, he points out that online comments on news items are a new genre that has come about as a consequence of developments in the interactive potential of newspaper websites. On the other hand, he selects two news reports out of a much larger set because they were at the top of a rank-ordered list based on the number of readers' comments on each article.

Ethical issues are also a crucial consideration in selecting an online source of data. If you are considering a study in this area, Chapter 3 provides a detailed account of the different ethical challenges that apply to different contexts and kinds of data. Online comments on news articles, for example, are anonymous, publicly accessible, and part of a general discussion of a particular topic, and therefore can generally be used for research purposes without asking for permission from the authors, although you are still likely to have to submit an ethics application (Collins, 2019). In the case of online health advice columns, in contrast, there are both issues of consent and of access to data. For all three studies discussed in this chapter that investigated online advice for young people, users of the site give permission for their messages to be used for research purposes at the point of registration (Locher, 2006, Harvey, 2012, Mullany et al., 2015). In all cases, requests for advice are also anonymous and the researchers contacted the site owners to inform them about the research. In two cases (Harvey, 2012, Mullany et al., 2015), the data was even provided by the site owners. In the case of Baker et al.'s (2019) study of patients' online feedback on NHS services in England, the researchers were in fact approached by the site owners and asked to investigate specific questions about the online feedback. Chapter 3 gives some further guidance on how data provided by an external organization in this way can be approached, in terms of ethics as well as data protection laws.

As mentioned in Chapter 3, unless your project is part of a wider research programme where ethical approval is granted to a whole team, it is advisable to focus on online data sources that are publicly accessible (i.e. can be read by any-one without having to register) and where users consent to their contributions being used for research purposes before they can post on the relevant website. Even in these cases, it can be appropriate to seek consent from the site owners and to comply with any additional requirements they may have.

7.2.2 Handling large data quantities

As we have already mentioned, online data is potentially available in very large quantities. In this chapter, we will therefore foreground the ways in which dif-ferent studies handle large data sources and large datasets (see also Chapters 2 and 11).

Locher (2006), for example, collects 2,286 question-answer pairs from a University online health advice column, i.e. all of the material that had been posted on that column up to the point of data collection in 2004. As the ques-tion-answer pairs are organized under seven topic categories (e.g. 'emotional health', 'sexual health'), she then selects 40 pairs for each topic category for the purposes of detailed analysis:

> a subcorpus was compiled with 40 records from each topic category. This corresponds to 12 percent of the entire corpus. I used the length of the answers as a criterion for inclusion. I established how many records occur within every window of 100 words and then calculated the percentage. As a second step, I randomly chose the corresponding number of records for the sub corpus. In other words, I tried to imitate the distribution of answers in each topic category by choosing a proportional number of records per 100 word steps. In this way, I obtained a sample of answers that is as repre-sentative as possible for each topic category.
>
> *(Locher, 2006: 15)*

The resulting collection of 280 question-answer pairs is then analyzed quali-tatively, for example in terms of advice-giving strategies. Nonetheless, as the smaller sub-set was selected randomly for each topic, the quantitative observa-tions that Locher makes can be more confidently generalized to the entire dataset than if they had been selected because they exemplify the phenomena that the researcher is interested in.

Most of the studies discussed in this chapter employ corpus linguistic methods to analyze large datasets, and also involve the principled selection of small sam-ples of data for detailed analysis.

7.3 Selected studies

In this section we show how it is possible to study the language of online health advice interactions to gain insights into the challenges, strategies and experiences of both advice-givers and advice-seekers. We then move on to looking at different types of user-generated comments on health-related news articles and health services.

7.3.1 Challenges and opportunities in providing expert health advice online

Studying the language used by those who act as online experts on health-related matters can provide insights into how they negotiate the challenges and opportunities of acting in that role. These include, for example, establishing a relationship with those who ask for advice and providing answers that are simultaneously appropriate for an individual questioner and for the much wider audience who may consult the relevant website. In this section, we discuss two specific studies that focus on data from, respectively, China and the USA.

Empathy in doctor-patient interactions is well-known to be an important factor in patient-centred care and patient satisfaction (Bonvicini et al., 2009, Howick et al., 2018). However, Zhang (2021) points out that research on empathy in healthcare settings has mainly focused on face-to-face interactions (Pounds, 2010; see also Chapter 6) or, when considering online interactions, Western contexts (Pounds, 2018). Zhang therefore explores the pragmatic functions of doctors' expressions of empathy in a selection of interactions on one of China's top five online healthcare platforms, '*Chunyu* Doctor'. This study is made particularly relevant by the role that online medical communication is increasingly playing in China to address a gap between supply and demand in healthcare services.

Zhang draws from previous studies to identify (a) patients' expressions of negative emotions, whether explicit (e.g. 'I'm very worried') or implicit (e.g. 'A family member passed away back home'), and (b) doctors' empathic responses to such expressions of negative emotions. The latter can involve acknowledging the patient's feelings (e.g. 'I can understand your feeling'), legitimizing or sharing those feelings (e.g. 'You are right to be worried') and providing a positive evaluation (e.g. 'The child is ill, and you family members have done your best') (Zhang, 2021: 818).

A sample of 100 asynchronous text-based interactions were then analyzed, drawn from an archive that contains completed consultations which were made publicly available for others' benefit, after receiving individual consent from the patients involved. The analysis reveals that empathic responses provided by doctors perform two main overarching functions: 'achieving a doctor's personal goals vis-à-vis his or her e-healthcare performance' and 'facilitating the institutional task of problem-solving' (Zhang, 2021: 818).

The former function is shown in Example 7.1 in the Introduction to this chapter: the use of 'we' and '[o]ur common goal' express empathy by aligning the doctor with the patient's personal perspective. This, Zhang argues, facilitates the doctor's next move, which is to encourage the patient to return with further questions in future and to post a positive comment on the website. Therefore, Zhang suggests, the preceding empathic talk could be argued to be produced in the ultimate service of self-promotion.

An example of the problem-solving function is the following extract from an interaction involving a 17-year-old patient with several tumours:

EXAMPLE 7.2

Doctor: Did your parents know about the illness?

Patient: Yes, they knew, but only about the tumor in my leg.
I was afraid they would get worried, if they knew about the tumors in other parts of my body. So I didn't tell them.

Doctor: Oh, you are strong and considerate in your fear that your parents will get worried [three thumbs up emojis].
Do you have a cough? (Zhang, 2021: 821)

Here, Zhang points out, the doctor provides a positive evaluation of the patient's explicitly expressed concern about her parents ('you are strong and considerate in your fear … ' and the thumbs up emojis) to mitigate the potential abruptness of a request for further information about a specific symptom that had not previously been mentioned ('Do you have a cough?').

This study provides a good opportunity to mention the reporting of examples in languages other than the one in which your research is reported. Zhang does not provide Mandarin originals for extracts from the data, but states in a note that they are available on request. Generally speaking, if you are conducting or publishing your research in, for example, an English speaking context, the gold standard is to provide examples in the original language, followed by a translation into English (see Chapter 8 for an example of how this can be done).

Overall, Zhang (2021) points out that it is possible that textual manifestations of empathy in written online medical interactions might partly make up for the lack of the expressive cues that are possible in spoken, and especially face-to-face, interactions. More generally, this study is presented as a contribution to a greater understanding of a the growing phenomenon of digitally mediated healthcare provision, and of its challenges and affordances for both doctors and patients.

Locher (2006, 2010) studied an online health advice column run by a University in the USA for the benefit of students. The University is referred to anonymously as AEI ('American Educational Institution'), and the column as 'Lucy Answers'. At the time of data collection in the mid-2000s, the site received over 2,000 questions a week, on topics organized into seven main categories, including 'alcohol and drugs', 'general health', 'sexual health', and 'emotional health'. Five questions were answered publicly by a team of health educators under the joint pseudonym 'Lucy', preserving the anonymity of advice-seekers. Locher collected from the web-archive of Lucy Answers all the material that was posted up to March 2004. This amounted to 2,286 question-answer sequences, for a total of 990,036 words. From this relatively large corpus, Locher selected a sample of 280 question-answer sequences – 40 for each of the 7 topic categories, for a total of 119,866 words (see above for her approach to randomized selection). These were then analyzed qualitatively for several different phenomena, a selection of which will be discussed here.

Among Locher's concerns are the linguistic strategies that are used in Lucy Answers to manage two potential challenges in providing online health advice to anonymous individuals on a public website: how to balance the provision of detailed information, including about a potential diagnosis, without being able to ask for further information; and how to signal a personal relationship with the individual questioner while also taking into account the wider audience for whom each answer is meant to be relevant.

Let's take as an example a response to a student who asked for advice about whether a virus they had picked up from their roommate could be 'mono', i.e. mononucleosis (Locher, 2010: 48–50). The lengthiest and central part of Lucy's answer to this particular question consists of an overview of mononucleosis, which begins as follows:

EXAMPLE 7.3

> Infectious mononucleosis (or mono) is caused by the Epstein-Barr virus. In developed countries, where individuals are not exposed as children, the peak years for mono infection are fourteen to eighteen (most adults are probably immune). The period during which mono is contagious is not completely clear. Most people with mono don't know where or from whom they got it.
>
> *(Locher, 2010: 48)*

As Locher points out, this kind of explanation is characterized by the use of technical terms (e.g. 'Epstein-Barr virus') and general information that goes beyond the specific concerns of the individual questioner (e.g. 'In developed countries … '). Indeed, the response then goes on to provide generic information about symptoms, the relevance of medication, the usual progression of the disease, and the complications that can arise in rare cases. This section of the response, Locher argues, has the dual purpose to reinforce the writer's expert credentials and to provide general information that may be relevant to anybody who might search the website to find out about mononucleosis.

In contrast, the beginning and end of the response are tailored to the specific individual questioner:

EXAMPLE 7.4

> (Beginning) Dear Curious,
> Lucy definitely can't diagnose your friend's illness through your letter, but his symptoms do not appear to match mono.

(End) If you continue to feel okay, you probably don't have much to worry about _ even when your roommate returns.

In both cases, Locher points out the presence of 'mitigation' strategies with regard to the advice. At the beginning, we have a 'disclaimer' ('Lucy definitely can't diagnose … '), defined as 'a move that demonstrates that not enough background information is given in order to properly diagnose the condition' (Locher, 2010: 49). At the end, an 'if clause' spells out a condition that needs to be satisfied at the advice-seeker's end ('if you continue to feel ok') for the applicability of the advice that follows in the main clause ('you probably don't have much to worry about'). By analyzing her dataset systematically, Locher found that 'if clauses' were routinely used in this way, as the responder has no way to obtain additional information from the advice-seeker, in contrast to traditional or, at any rate, interactional medical consultations. In Locher's data, the 'if clause' preceded the main clause in the majority of cases, which she takes as evidence that '*Lucy* prefers to establish relevance for her readers as soon as possible' (Locher, 2006: 98). This also shifts the ultimate responsibility for whether the advice applies or not onto the advice-seekers themselves. Locher additionally points out that the giving of advice (whether online or in face-to-face situations) involves an imbalance of expertise and, in some cases, power that can threaten the advice-seeker's face, i.e. their public image as a competent and independent person (Goffman, 1967; Brown & Levinson, 1987; see Chapters 2 and 6). Mitigation strategies such as disclaimers and hedges reduce the asymmetry between advice-giver and advice-seeker, and therefore decrease this potential face threat.

Relatedly, Locher (2006) considers how Lucy Answers manages the interpersonal challenge of simultaneously addressing an individual and a wider audience. The personal dimension is handled, for example, by comments that show empathy for the specific advice-seeker, and therefore establish a connection with them:

EXAMPLE 7.5

You are not alone in feeling shy – although it probably feels that way.

(Locher, 2006: 180)

At the same time, answers can also explicitly address a broader audience who may share similar concerns, as in 'You and everyone else at AEI' and 'For those of you unfamiliar with … ' (Locher, 2006: 181). Similarly, a categorization of the titles of responses shows that they are formulated in ways that signal their broad relevance, for example by means of 'neutral subject headings from which the reader can immediately infer the topic of the record', such as 'Marijuana and driving', 'Aspirin therapy', and 'Alcohol use and memory loss' (Locher, 2006: 157).

Locher uses the findings of her analyses as the basis for recommending to healthcare professionals the benefits of online advice columns, which she summarizes as follows:

(1)   Availability and anonymity;
(2)   Personal appeal, identification potential;
(3)   Possibility of reaching many with a 'personalized' response;
(4)   Possibility of adapting the text to the needs of the target group;
(5)   The archive and hyperlinking. (Locher, 2010: 51)

The studies we discuss in the next section make similar points about the advantages of online advice sites, particularly for teenagers. In addition, the next section shows in more detail how the use of corpus linguistic methods makes it possible to combine quantitative and qualitative analyses of large datasets.

7.3.2 Adolescents' concerns on a dedicated health advice website

Studying the language used to ask for health-related advice online can provide insights into people's concerns and experiences that may not be easy to obtain otherwise, and in turn reveal the role that online advice sources can play in people's lives. Both of the studies we discuss in this section combine corpus linguistic methods with discourse analysis to explore adolescents' health concerns as expressed on the UK-based website 'Teenage Health Freak'. Below is an example of a message that was sent to the website's 'Virtual Surgery' via its electronic messaging facility (a kind of anonymous email service) by a 13-year-old female advice-seeker:

EXAMPLE 7.6

> I want to look anorexic. I know its really 'stupid,' but i like the idea of being able to see my bones. I've started restricting my calorie intake to around 650 a day, and eating mostly negative calorie foods. Also i CandS (Chew and spit) and i've tried purging (but for some reason i can't do it). what's going on with me. I feel stupid for wanting to look like that because i know its dangerous, but i want it.
>
> *(Mullany et al., 2015: 220)*

Mullany et al. (2015) comment that this message exemplifies the consequences, for teenagers, of a prevailing 'discourse of slenderness', as well as a tension between anorexia as a disorder ('i know it's dangerous') and anorexia as a lifestyle choice ('I want to look anorexic').

Example 7.6 is one of 113,480 requests for advice about weight and eating that were analyzed by Mullany et al. (2015), for a total of approximately 2 million words, while Harvey (2012) studied 62,794 messages about mental health problems, for a total of approximately 1 million words. Similarly to Locher (2010), both studies emphasize the importance for adolescents to be able to seek advice about potentially sensitive and embarrassing topics through anonymous online environments, and the opportunities afforded by such anonymous requests for advice to investigate the concerns and lived experience of teenagers. From the perspective of ethics, as we mentioned earlier, users of the electronic messaging facility on Teenage Health Freak are informed that their messages may be used for research purposes, while guaranteeing anonymity. In addition, Harvey (2012: 355), who is also a co-author in Mullany et al. (2015) spells out that the website operators gave permission for the study to be conducted, and provided the data that was analyzed.

Mullany et al. begin by carrying out a keyword analysis – a technique we describe in Chapter 3. The whole 2-million-word corpus from Teenage Health Freaks was compared to the 100-million-word British National Corpus as reference corpus. Mullany et al. employed Log Likelihood as statistical significance measure (the default option in the software WordSmith Tools at the time) with a threshold that corresponds to p <0.000001. This means that there is less than one chance in a million that the results could have occurred by chance.

This approach generated 2,000 keywords, which were then manually grouped according to the area of health that they related to. This resulted in five broad themes which reflect the main health concerns of the adolescents who seek advice from the website:

- Sex/Pregnancy/Relationships;
- Sexual Body Parts;
- Body Changes;
- Weight and Eating;
- Smoking/Drugs/Alcohol.

Out of these five themes, Mullany et al. select Weight and Eating for further analysis, as messages about this broad topic have the highest median length (19 words), which is taken as an indication that they go into greater detail than messages about the other topics.

The 40 keywords subsumed under Weight and Eating provide more detail regarding the areas where adolescents require health advice (e.g. 'anorexia', 'bulimia', 'dieting', 'vegan', 'exercise'). They also reveal the 'mixture of registers' that advice-seekers are able to employ (Mullany et al., 2015: 215), including, for example, technical medical terms (e.g. 'BMI', 'bulimic'), general health-related words (e.g. 'weight', 'diet'), and colloquial items (e.g. 'chubby', 'veggie').

Mullany et al. then focus more specifically on the types of questions that are asked about the topic of weight and eating. To do this, they consider all two-word clusters (also known in Corpus Linguistics as 'n-grams') in a sub-section of the corpus consisting of messages that contain at least one of the 40 relevant keywords. Among the two-word clusters, they identify those that are used to form questions:

- What is
- What should
- How do

- What do
- How can
- What can
- Why do
- What are
- What does

A manual analysis of ten-word chunks beginning with any of these question-forming clusters is used to identify the top ten types of question about Weight and eating. Half of these question types are to do with weight, as in the case of the question type *What is the average/normal weight for x?*, which captures examples such as 'What should my weight be?'. This is consistent with the earlier finding that 'anorexia'/'anorexic' and 'bulimia'/'bulimic' are among the top 20 keywords in the corpus as a whole. These observations lead to a further zooming in of the analysis to focus on the requests for advice that contain the words 'anorexia'/'anorexic', 'bulimia'/'bulimic', resulting in two more specific sub-sets of data: 430 messages about anorexia and 120 messages about bulimia.

At this point, a manual, qualitative analysis of these messages is both practically possible and required by Mullany et al.'s goal to classify them according to the precise topic of the request. The message we quoted at the beginning of this section, for example, is classified as belonging to a 'post diagnosis' group of messages, where the writer assumes that they have anorexia or bulimia (as opposed to messages classified as 'requests for diagnosis'). The example is cited specifically because it takes an 'anti-recovery perspective' (Fox et al., 2005), i.e. it expresses a desire to have an eating disorder, or, as we mentioned earlier, a tension between such a desire and an awareness of the dangers associated with eating disorders.

Overall, this study highlights the importance of online sources of anonymous health advice for adolescents, and the insights that can be achieved into their concerns and experiences by applying discourse analysis to this kind of data.

A similar approach to a 1-million-word corpus from the same website (62,794 messages) was adopted by Harvey (2012), but with a focus on mental health, and specifically depression. Harvey uses WordSmith tools and the same threshold for statistical significance as Mullany et al. (2015) to carry out a keyness comparison between this corpus and the 10-million-word spoken section of the British National Corpus, which consists of transcripts of both informal and formal speech from the mid-1990s (but note that a new version of the British National Corpus now exists (BNC2014), consisting mainly of data from the mid-2010s: http://corpora.lancs.ac.uk/bnc2014/). Harvey then divides the resulting 3,258 keywords into 12 thematic groupings. These include several of the groups identified by Mullany et al. (e.g. Body Weight, Drugs/alcohol), but also some additional groupings, and specifically Mental health (e.g. 'depression', 'suicide', 'self-harm', 'cry'), which is the focus of Harvey's study.

The similarities and differences between the keywords, and thematic groupings, in the two studies provide an opportunity to reflect further on this particular technique. The two studies involved messages collected from the Teenage Health Freaks website at different points in time. On the one hand, there is no reason to expect that they would involve radically different concerns on the part of the senders of the requests for advice, and indeed, there are many shared keywords and grouping across the two studies. On the other hand, it is of course possible that concerns changed over time, which could itself be a topic for investigation. From a methodological perspective, however, it is important to notice that the two studies use different reference corpora: Mullany et al. use the whole of the 100-million-words British National Corpus while Harvey uses the 10-million-word spoken section. Although it has been found that the results of keyness analyses are remarkably stable across different comparisons (Scott, 1999), this is a useful reminder that keyness analyses are comparative, and that the choice of reference corpus can affect one's results. In this case, the presence of a Mental health grouping in Harvey's results but not in Mullany et al.'s may suggests that the whole of the British National Corpus included enough references to mental health and illness for those terms not to be identified as keywords in that comparison, in contrast with the spoken section only.

Having decided to study messages about mental health in his corpus, Harvey points out that 'depressed' and 'depression' are by far the most frequent keywords in the relevant grouping, and therefore focuses on those two terms specifically. He then employs the corpus linguistic technique of collocation analysis (see Chapter 2) to identify the words that tend to occur with distinctively high frequencies in close proximity to 'depressed' and 'depression'. This enables him to notice, for example, that both words tend to collocate with the first-person singular pronouns 'I' and 'me', suggesting that adolescents tend to write for advice about their own personal experiences around depression rather than other people's, such as friends or family members. In addition, the collocation analysis shows that, not surprisingly, 'depressed' collocates with 'am', while 'depression' collocates with 'have'. Harvey then considers in detail the concordance lines for 'I am depressed' and 'I have depression', to investigate differences between these two structures and the kind of requests for advice that they tend to be part of.

The analysis of concordance lines reveals that 'depressed' in 'I am depressed' tends to be used in a relatively loose sense to refer to negative emotional states that are presented as the consequence of something that is explicitly mentioned in the message, such as problems with romantic relationships or friendship groups:

EXAMPLE 7.7

I'm really depressed about splitting up with my boyfriend. I still like him and its getting me down.

EXAMPLE 7.8

> i am not happy with myself i am fat i get bullied and i am depressed
>
> *(Harvey, 2012: 363)*

As a consequence, 'I am depressed' tends to be found in messages that ask for advice about the *cause* of the negative feelings rather than the negative feelings themselves. In these messages, 'depressed' therefore seems to capture an experience that is presented as context-bound and transient.

In contrast, Harvey points out that 'I have depression' tends to be used in a more technical sense to refer to a diagnosis that has either been formally received by the advice-seeker or that, minimally, the advice-seeker thinks applies to them:

EXAMPLE 7.9

> I have depression, and it seems to be getting worse lately. i've been feeling horrible through most of the hols, and i still do even though im back at school. i was thinking of dropping out, but ive decided to stay and drop a subject instead. but how can i make myself feel better? i'm putting my family through a lot of grief.

EXAMPLE 7.10

> dear Dr Ann, i have had depression since the age of 11/12 but have never spoken to anyone about it. recently this depression has got to me more and I have started cuttin my wrist … with some intent to kill myself. At good times i don't want to do this so is there anything i can do to prevent it happening next time i have another long spell of depression?

As such, the messages that include 'I have depression' tend to be associated with a clinical, potentially pathologizing view of negative emotional states, which seem to be perceived as a relatively stable characteristic of the person that they have little control over. In these cases, what is sought is advice on how to handle the *consequences* of the depression.

Overall, like Mullany et al. (2015), Harvey emphasizes the importance of detailed analysis of adolescents' own spontaneous ways of referring to and describing their own experiences. In this particular study, this reveals different views of what may be referred to as 'being depressed' or 'depression', and their consequences for the person's own sense of self. In both studies, corpus linguistic methods make it possible to begin with a broad overview of the data, move on to focus on patterns and expressions that are particularly distinctive or frequent, and finally to analyze examples in their context of use, which leads to nuanced observations about people's use of language and underlying experiences.

In the next section we turn to the analysis of comments that are posted publicly online on, respectively, health-related news reports and the services provided by the National Health Service in England. This will also involve the use of corpus linguistic techniques that we have not discussed so far.

7.3.3 Readers' perceptions of a global health threat in online comments on news reports

In Chapter 4 we discussed a corpus-based study of news reports on the topic of Antimicrobial Resistance (AMR) – the increasing emergence of strains of bacterial diseases that do not respond to existing antibiotics. Here we focus on a related study by Collins (2019) that aimed to understand people's attitudes about AMR by studying online comments on news reports about the implications of AMR for some sexually transmitted diseases that are normally treated with antibiotics.

The possibility for readers to comment on online news reports has created valuable opportunities to study the reception of and engagement with news items on the part of the public. For our purposes, this is of course relevant when the news is health related.

Collins (2019) created a corpus consisting of all articles published in 2017 in UK national newspapers that contained at least one of three expressions: 'AMR', 'antibiotic resistant', 'antibiotic resistance'. He then manually ranked the articles in the corpus by the number of readers' comments they received on the relevant newspaper's website, and selected two out of the top three highest ranked articles for detailed analysis. These were the top ranked article, from the MailOnline, and the third highest ranked article, from the Guardian. The latter was chosen in preference to the second ranked article, because it related to the same WHO press release about an antibiotic-resistant strain of the sexually transmitted disease gonorrhoea. An additional reason for selecting articles from these two newspapers is that they contrast in political orientation – an important consideration when comparing different news outlets – with the Guardian being located towards the left of the political spectrum and the MailOnline (the online version of the Daily Mail) towards the right.

The MailOnline article elicited 1,883 comments (amounting to 24,947 words) while the Guardian article elicited 835 comments (amounting to 23,355 words). To analyze this data, Collins conducted keyness analyses at the level of semantic domains, rather than at the word level (Rayson, 2008). Each article and set of comments were compared to the same reference corpus (the one-million-word Written Sampler of the British National Corpus) by means of the USAS Semantic Annotation tool in the online software Wmatrix (Rayson, 2008). The USAS tagger in Wmatrix allocates each word in an uploaded corpus to one of 21 major discourse fields (e.g. 'The body and the individual'), which are in turn divided into 232 semantic fields or domains (e.g. 'Medicines and medical treatment', which is subsumed under 'The body and the individual' and is applied to lexical items such as 'antibiotics').

Keyness analyses at the level of semantic domains have two main advantages. They may reveal patterns that are missed by word-level comparisons when the patterns involve words that have similar meanings (e.g. 'antibiotic', 'antibiotics', 'antibacterial', 'antimicrobial'), but that are not sufficiently overused, individually, to appear as keywords. Moreover, because each semantic domain includes many different words, the analyst tends to have to deal with a smaller, and therefore more manageable, number of results. For example, in Collins' study, a word-level comparison of MailOnline comments with the reference corpus generated 386 results, but a comparison at the level of semantic domains generated 29 results, based on the same statistical measures.

For both newspapers, Collins compares the article and the comments with the same reference corpus. He then establishes which semantic domains are key both in the article and its own set of comments and which are only key in one or the other. This answers the question: do commenters overuse the same semantic fields that are overused in the articles that they are commenting on?

For the Guardian, all of the semantic domains that were found to be key in the article were also found to be key in the comments. These were to do with sexual behaviours, health, medicine, and illness. In addition, even though AMR was only briefly mentioned in the article itself, it was referred to in the comments often enough for two relevant semantic domains to be key: Living creatures (including the words 'bacteria' and 'superbug') and Helping/hindering (including 'resistance') (Collins, 2019: 163). For the MailOnline, in contrast, there were differences as well as overlaps in the respective sets of key semantic domains. The shared key semantic domains between the article and comments were to do with sexual behaviours, physiology, health, illness, and treatment. However, none of the key semantic domains that, in the article, contained words relating to the rise and dangers of AMR were found to be key in the comments. On the other hand, there were additional key domains in the MailOnline comments that were not key in the article. These were to do with sexual habits and behaviours, and the extent to which the pleasures of sex are worth running the risks that may be associated with it.

In other words, Collins' analysis shows that commenters on the MailOnline article reacted more to the specific example of a sexually transmitted disease than to the more general issue of AMR, and engaged in more detailed discussions about personal and moral issues to do with different kinds of sexual behaviour than the article did. This finding provides further evidence of relatively low levels of concern about the dangers of AMR among some sections of the public, and therefore has potential implications for public health campaigns aimed at increasing awareness and changing behaviours in relation to antibiotics use.

7.3.4 Patients' online feedback on health services

In some cases, research on language and health is carried out in response to questions that come directly from stakeholders in healthcare (we discuss different inspirations for research questions in Chapter 11 too). This was the case for a study by Baker et al. (2019) on comments posted by patients on the NHS Choices website – where the National Health Service in England provides an opportunity to users of their services to give feedback on their experiences. Below are two examples of such comments:

EXAMPLE 7.11

> I received the best treatment I could have wished for. Everyone was extremely polite and caring and made me feel at ease.
>
> *(Baker et al., 2019: 46)*

EXAMPLE 7.12

> Poor poor poor I've been at this surgery for a number of years and there's not been one time when I ever felt my doctor or any of their locums were actually interested in what was wrong with me. The reception staff aren't much better, I guess they take their lead from the top.
>
> *(Baker et al., 2019: 50)*

It is a common practice, in healthcare systems throughout the world, to collect feedback from patients in various forms, from written questionnaires to telephone surveys. This practice has the potential to empower patients and drive service improvements based on their experiences, but it is also a reflection of a neoliberal tendency and a deliberate drive in some parts of the world to emphasize choice in healthcare and to view patients as consumers. In practice, the feedback can be used by organizations such as the NHS to lobby government for additional funding, based on good performance or evidence of unmet needs, but also to conduct performance-related interventions at different levels of organizational structure, as well as to reduce or divert funding in case of perceptions of underperformance (Brookes & Baker, 2017).

In the case of the NHS Choices website, patients provide feedback via a 5-point scale from one to five stars and, if they wish, by adding a comment (such as the ones above) in a free-text box. In the mid-2010s, this posed a challenge for the Feedback team at NHS England. While they could easily gather and analyze the numerical feedback given via the star system, the free-text option generated so much textual material that it could not be analyzed manually. A team at Lancaster University led by Paul Baker was therefore commissioned to analyze the data by employing corpus-based methods (Brookes & Baker, 2017, Baker et al., 2019).

The team constructed a corpus consisting of all comments posted on the NHS Choices website from March 2013 to September 2015. This amounted to 228,113 comments and approximately 29 million words. The comments related to different kinds of NHS services, but the majority were to do with GP practices, hospitals, and dentists. The analysis was guided by 12 questions formulated by NHS England, of which the most general was: 'What are the key drivers for positive and negative feedback?'

The first step in the analysis was to extract a frequency list from the corpus (a rank-ordered list with the most frequent words at the top), and identify the most frequent words that suggest evaluation. This led to the compilation of two lists consisting of the 10 most frequent words that express positive evaluation and the 10 most frequent words that express negative evaluation:

> Positive evaluation: 'good', 'excellent', 'great', 'best', 'fantastic', 'brilliant', 'wonderful', 'amazing', 'outstanding', 'exceptional'.
>
> Negative evaluation: 'bad', 'poor', 'worst', 'worse', 'terrible', 'awful', 'appalling', 'joke', 'disgusting', 'ridiculous'.
>
> *(Baker et al., 2019: 41)*

Overall, the positive words are approximately three times more frequent than the negative words (223,439 cumulative occurrences vs. 74,304), suggesting a general bias towards positive evaluation in the corpus.

It should be born in mind that the most frequent words in a corpus are different from the keywords in a corpus. Keywords are words that are *overused* as compared with a reference corpus, but they may not be among the most frequent words in a corpus. In turn, highly frequent words in a corpus may not be key in a particular comparison if they have similar relative frequencies in the reference corpus. The above lists also show that decisions about what counted as a positive or negative evaluation word needed to take into account how the word is used in the dataset in question. For example, 'joke' – the only noun in the lists above – was found to be used in expressions such as 'What a joke', which suggest negative evaluation.

Having identified the most common ways of expressing evaluation in the data, the second step in the analysis was to compute the collocates of each of the 20 adjectives, and group them thematically to capture the main areas of NHS services that were the topic of the feedback. Brookes and Baker (2017) summarize the findings of this stage of the analysis as follows:

> Four areas emerged as frequent across the comments (corresponding words in brackets): (1) treatment (*care, treatment, dental*); (2) communication (*communication, attention, listener(s), advice*); (3) interpersonal skills (*atmosphere, attitude(s), manner(s)*) and (4) system/organisation (*system, appointment, management, waiting time(s)*).
>
> *(Brookes & Baker, 2017: 4)*

Of these four areas, two were evaluated positively in the largest proportion of cases: treatment (87%) and communication (77%). In contrast, interpersonal skills and system/organizational issues were evaluated positively in less than half of cases: 44% and 41% respectively. Crucially, however, an examination of concordance lines for the collocates of all 20 evaluative words showed that the interpersonal skills of staff were the most frequent reason for providing either positive and negative feedback (accounting for approximately 40% of cases; Baker et al., 2019: 43–9).

In view of these findings, let's reconsider Examples 11 and 12 above. Example 7.11 shows that, even when the feedback is explicitly concerned with treatment, the person comments positively on the attitude that the staff had towards them ('extremely polite and caring'). Example 7.12 is one of 200 comments that Baker et al. (2019) analyzed in detail because they contained sequences of at least two occurrences of 'poor' (150 comments had two successive occurrences of the word and 50 had three, as in this case). Of these 200 comments, 66% were about staff interpersonal skills. In both cases, the writer mentions how they 'felt' as a consequence of the attitude of the staff, and include different kinds of health professionals (cf. 'everyone' in Example 7.11 and 'my doctor', 'any of their locums' and 'reception staff' in Example 7.12).

Receptionists in particular were found to be the fourth most frequently mentioned category of NHS staff in the comments (after doctors/GPs, dentists and nurses) (Baker et al., 2019: 100), and were also the group that received the least positive evaluations. An examination of collocational pairs between references to different staff groups and the 20 evaluative words mentioned earlier showed that receptionists were evaluated positively in 57% of cases, in contrast with, for example, over 90% for dentists, surgeons, and paramedics. When receptionists were criticized, the focus was inevitably on interpersonal skills and communication. An examination of 100 comments that included the word 'receptionist' and were associated with a low star rating (one or two stars) revealed that, in 18 cases, the receptionist was described as 'rude' and, in 40 additional cases, via an adjective similarly suggesting a negative attitude towards the patient (e.g. 'aggressive', 'dismissive', 'unpleasant') or behaviours such as shouting (Baker et al., 2019: 107).

However, Baker et al. (2019:) point out that receptionists at GP practices are regularly criticized for doing what is in fact required by their triaging role, i.e. for asking questions about the reasons why someone wants to be seen by a doctor:

EXAMPLE 7.13

> My daughter is now too embarrassed to go back when she was asked personal questions about the nature of her ailment by the receptionist.
>
> *(Baker et al., 2019: 109)*

One way of interpreting this pattern, therefore, is that some of the least well-paid and least prestigious roles within the organization, who are also overwhelmingly female, attract the most criticism for doing their job in difficult circumstances, especially considering that demand for appointments usually exceeds availability.

As with the corpus-based studies discussed in the previous section, the initial keyness analysis made it possible to identify distinctive words and topic areas in the corpus as a whole. By focusing on some of those words and topic areas, Baker et al. (2019) were then able to zoom into datasets that were small enough to be analyzed manually, and to select representative examples for detailed discussion of how individuals make use of the opportunities provided by the NHS Choices website.

On the basis of their findings, Baker and colleagues recommend that NHS England increases its focus on staff interpersonal skills, both in terms of training and of creating environments that are conducive to the delivery of patient-centred care (e.g. by making sure that staff have enough time to treat patients as individuals). Crucially, this focus should involve *all* staff groups, including those in administrative roles, such as receptionists. More generally, Baker and colleagues emphasize the importance of a systematic understanding of the concerns expressed in patients' feedback as a basis for improvements in services.

7.4 Concluding remarks

Digital communication through a variety of online environments provides new opportunities for health-related advice-seeking/giving and for patients and the public to comment on health-related topics and services. Linguistic approaches to such online communication can achieve important insights into people's health-related concerns and experiences, highlight the challenges of providing health advice online and provide evidence that is relevant to public health campaigns and improvements in health services. As we have shown, research in this area often combines quantitative and qualitative analysis, including particularly by exploiting corpus linguistic techniques. The final chapter in Part II of this book will provide further examples of how corpus and other methods can be used to investigate different aspects of digital health communication.

Further readings

Brookes, G., & Baker, P. (2022). Cancer services patient experience in England: Quantitative and qualitative analyses of the National Cancer Patient Experience Survey. *BMJ Supportive and Palliative Care*, 1–7.

Mao, Y., & Zhao, X. (2019). I am a doctor, and here is my proof: Chinese doctors' identity constructed on the online medical consultation Websites. *Health Communication*, *34*(13), 1645–1652. https://doi.org/10.1080/10410236.2018.1517635

Pounds, G., & De Pablos-Ortega, C. (2016). Patient-centred communication in British, Italian and Spanish Ask-the-Expert healthcare websites. *Communication and Medicine*, *12*(2–3), 225–241.

References

Baker, P., Brookes, G., & Evans, C. (2019). *The language of patient feedback: A corpus linguistic study of online health communication*. Routledge.

Bonvicini, K. A., Perlin, M. J., Bylund, C. L., Carroll, G., Rouse, R. A., & Goldstein, M. G. (2009). Impact of communication training on physician expression of empathy in patient encounters. *Patient Education and Counseling*, *75*(1), 3–10.

Brookes, G., & Baker, P. (2017). What does patient feedback reveal about the NHS? A mixed methods study of comments posted to the NHS Choices online service. *BMJ Open*, *7*(4), E013821.

Brown, P., & Levinson, S. C. (1987). *Politeness: Some universals in language use*. Cambridge University Press.

Collins, L. (2019). *Corpus linguistics for online communication: A guide for research*. Routledge.

Fox, N., Ward, K., & O'Rourke, A. (2005). Proanorexia, weight-loss drugs and the internet: An 'anti-recovery' explanatory model of anorexia. *Sociology of Health and Illness*, 27(7), 944–971.

Goffman, E. (1967). *Interaction ritual: Essays on face-to-face interaction*. Aldine Publishing.

Harvey, K. (2012). Disclosures of depression: Using corpus linguistics methods to examine young people's online health concerns. *International Journal of Corpus Linguistics*, 17(3), 349–379.

Howick, J., Moscrop, A., Mebius, A., Fanshawe, T. R., Lewith, G., Bishop, F. L., Mistiaen, P., Roberts, N. W., Dieninytė, E., Hu, X-Y., Aveyard, P., & Onakpoya, I. J. (2018). Effects of empathic and positive communication in healthcare consultations: A systematic review and meta-analysis. *Journal of the Royal Society of Medicine*, 111(7), 240–252.

Locher, M. (2006). *Advice online: Advice-giving in an American Internet health column*. John Benjamins.

Locher, M. A. (2010). Health Internet sites: A linguistic perspective on health advice columns. *Social Semiotics*, 20(1), 43–59.

Mullany, L., Smith, C., Harvey, K., & Adolphs, S. (2015). 'Am I anorexic?' weight, eating and discourses of the body in online adolescent health communication. *Communication and Medicine*, 12(2–3), 211–223.

O'Riordan, L. (2010). Ten vital things every woman needs to know about breast cancer. *The Mail on Sunday*. Retrieved October 9, 2022, from https://www.dailymail.co.uk/health/article-6146233/Breast-cancer-things-woman-needs-know-breast-surgeon-whos-twice.html

Pounds, G. (2010). Empathy as 'appraisal': A new language-based approach to the exploration of clinical empathy. *Journal of Applied Linguistics & Professional Practice*, 7(2), 139–162.

Pounds, G. (2018). Patient-centred communication in ask-the-expert healthcare websites. *Applied Linguistics*, 39, 117–134.

Rayson, P. (2008). From key words to key semantic domains. *International Journal of Corpus Linguistics*, 13(4), 519–549.

Scott, M. (1999). *WordSmith tools help manual*. Version 3.0. Mike Scott and Oxford University Press.

Wang, X., Shi, J., & Kong, H. (2021). Online health information seeking: A review and meta-analysis. *Health Communication*, 36(10), 1163–1175.

Zhang, Y. (2021). How doctors do things with empathy in online medical consultations in China: A discourse-analytic approach. *Health Communication*, 36(7), 816–825.

8

DIGITAL HEALTH COMMUNICATION AND THE LIVED EXPERIENCE OF ILLNESS

8.1 Introduction

As we discussed in the previous chapter, study after study has shown that the vast majority of Internet users turn to an online search engine after receiving an illness diagnosis. As in the studies outlined in Chapter 7, this can be to research symptoms and treatment options, to interact directly with health professionals online whether these are real licenced professionals or not, or indeed to provide or search for ratings and feedback on available healthcare services. Another way that people might use the Internet for health-related information and communication is by turning to online peer-to-peer forums where they can connect, interact with, or simply share and read stories by people who have relevant illnesses or healthcare experiences. As we noted in Chapter 5, such personal accounts provide insights into the lived experience of being ill and using healthcare that are crucially important not just for understanding and empathy, but also for sensitive and effective diagnosis, support, and treatment in the types of interactions patients have with healthcare professionals, discussed in Chapter 6. Of course, there are a number of channels for people to share their illness experiences. Before the digital age this could be via published memoirs, diaries, local support groups, or columns in a newspaper. Nowadays much of this is online whether via (micro) blogs, videos or indeed online fora. And it is well documented that sharing, but also just reading such experiences, has real health benefits (Cepeda et al., 2008).

Let's begin with a few examples from Demjén (2016) of the kinds of interactions that might happen on an online forum with peers, with similar experiences to oneself. These examples come from an online peer-to-peer forum that is part of the website of a cancer charity, so the forum itself is dedicated to experiences of cancer. The particular thread hosting this excerpt is mostly used by people with different forms of colorectal cancer and is entitled 'For those with a

DOI: 10.4324/9781003020417-10

warped sense of humour WARNING- no punches pulled here', or 'Warped' for short. Original spellings have been retained.

EXAMPLE 8.1

It's just one of the evil Mr Crab's funny little jokes that we now have to spend our lives thinking not just "What shall I have for tea?" but "What shall I have for this random nameless meal – that I am having at an odd time because I couldn't face food till now – that won't kill me?" I am pretty sure that my own evil Mr Crab has taken control of my stomach-to-brain signals. He gets hungry in the night, and demands steak and chips. I don't eat meat!! Bastard.

(Valerie)

EXAMPLE 8.2

we all know how Mr crab likes to fuck with you head and your body.

(emerald22)

EXAMPLE 8.3

of course all of us may not get there [to a ball] on the night due to a party pooper Mr Cancer who sometimes buggers up one's plans

(HoneyBee)

As Examples 8.1–8.3 show, contributors to this particular thread sometimes refer to cancer using the title 'Mr' and describe it as having independent traits, personalities, motivations, and behaviours. In other words, people personify their disease.

So why might people write about cancer in this way and what implications could it have? On the one hand, personifying cancer allows contributors to externalize their illness – separate it from themselves – and 'blame' the uncontrollable physical changes (e.g. to appetite) on 'someone' else. This potentially helps them to maintain a coherent sense of self in the face of rapid physical change and can be seen as a way of regaining some control over their situation. Perhaps more importantly, by jointly developing and engaging in this specific type of humorous lived experience representation, contributors to this thread become united through a shared language (just like in offline spaces) (Coates, 2007). Simply by using language in a particular way, you become part of a community. This sense of belonging has been described as a significant advantage of peer-to-peer health fora (e.g. Galegher et al., 1998; Patsos, 2001). Feeling like you 'have a tribe' is important in illness contexts where people can feel isolated and alone. The latter point is particularly true in the case of conditions or symptoms that are taboo (e.g. colorectal cancer, see below), rare (e.g. Takayasu arteritis, Patsos, 2001), or poorly delineated (e.g. post-natal depression, see below). One contributor on Warped even articulates the benefits of the online community for her offline life: 'you loony lot really did help me and I even laughed out loud in the Dr office […] I love you all, your my kinda folk.'

More broadly, first-hand accounts of illness and healthcare shared online can become invaluable sources of insider information for the general public when it comes to understanding what it feels like to be ill (i.e. in terms of Mischler's 'voice of the lifeworld' from Chapter 6), as well as being useful in medical education and practice. In this way, they can be similar to more formally published accounts, like those discussed in Chapter 5.

8.1.1 In this chapter

In this chapter we focus on digital interactions between peers, as well as less interactive instances of digital health discourse that might be found on YouTube or Facebook updates. In both cases, lived-experience accounts, or stories of personal experience, are presented and can be seen to perform multiple functions. We showcase studies that have explored how personal experiences on online health fora can be used for community building, what digital lived-experience accounts might reveal that is of relevance for medical practice, and how expertise and various identities can be performed on various online channels. The studies we review here mainly explore online fora, Facebook interactions, and YouTube videos, but similar studies can be carried out on blog posts, microblogs, Instagram posts, or any other digital platforms that have yet to be invented.

8.2 Preliminary considerations

As the above suggests, and as we have laid out in past chapters explicitly, all research projects, whatever their size, involve considerations that relate to deciding on the focus of analysis, the selection of data sources and/or recruitment of participants, the data quantity, the analytical tools, and ethics. Many of these are outlined in detail in Chapters 2 and 3. Here we focus specifically on what questions you might want to explore with digital data involving lived experience accounts and peer-to-peer interactions, and the kinds of approaches you might use to analyse these.

8.2.1 What kinds of questions to explore

The introductory examples above come from a large project funded by the UK's Economic and Social Research Council (grant number: ES/J007927/1), which, thanks to financial support, was able to explore multiple aspects of the data and publish several related studies on the basis of the same dataset. Very generally, all of these explored how language is used to communicate the experience of cancer and end-of-life care. As the examples above suggest, one particular study was interested in exploring what interpersonal and psychological functions might be performed by different aspects of language (parts-of-speech, metaphor, and humour) in an online peer-to-peer support forum. This is discussed in more detail in section 8.3.2. The second study in the same section (Stommel & Koole,

2010) used the tools of Conversation Analysis and membership categorization analysis to show that becoming part of a community is not a guaranteed outcome of interacting in an online support forum. Like the studies in section 8.3.1, you might also be interested in exploring the social reality of being ill. This could help you understand how social taboos might prevent some people (e.g. new mothers) from seeking and/or receiving the care they need. Alternatively, you might be more interested in more individual aspects of online lived-experience accounts, such as how they present or construct their writers and why, like the studies in section 8.3.3.

Other topics that have been studied with similar online data have been how lay-people tell their stories in ways that legitimize and support any advice they offer (Thurnherr et al., 2016) and how online forum users respond to expressions of uncertainty about medical interventions such as vaccines (see Chapter 11). And you can also look at how first-hand accounts online (whether interactive or not) might impact public perceptions of certain conditions or represent people with certain conditions, like you might do with the types of data discussed in Chapters 4 and 5.

8.2.2 Analytical tools

Similarly to the examples discussed in Chapter 7, the preliminary example above comes from a study that relied on corpus methods to enable a systematic analysis of more than 1.5 million words of data. As you will see in section 8.3.2, however, the same study also analyzed metaphor and humour, and could afford to spend time and effort on more qualitative case studies of individual lexical items or phrases. All these different analyses contribute to a more holistic picture of how language can be used to build online communities and, in some cases, to reframe or recast one's role in one's illness. Digital language data tends to be plentiful, so corpus linguistic tools can be very helpful. Semino et al. (2018) in section 8.3.2 use corpus tools to orient themselves within a very large dataset and to ensure that they focus on the most characteristic patterns. Coltman-Patel et al. (2022) and Kinloch and Jaworska (2020) in section 8.3.1 use the insights from corpus analyses as a spring-board or a way in to the data to investigating specific patterns in more detail. But that is not to say that corpus analysis is the only systematic means of approaching this kind of data.

The second study in section 8.3.2 for instance uses the qualitative and often quite time-intensive tools of Conversation Analysis and membership categorization analysis to understand how newcomers to an online support forum manage (or not) to become part of the community. This serves as a useful illustration that CA, which was originally developed for verbal interaction, can also be applied to written data as long as it is interactive (cf. Chapter 6). In section 8.3.3 Chou et al. (2011) use qualitative narrative analysis to explore what makes YouTube cancer stories authentic, while Koteyko and Hunt (2016) rely on digital ethnography to gain a range of sources of evidence for their analysis. In addition, other tools such as multimodal analysis (see Chapter 2 and 4) can also be very useful, depending on the type of data you have, including in combination with other lenses.

8.3 Selected studies

The rest of this chapter will cover personal experiences posted on online fora, social media platforms, and on YouTube.

8.3.1 *Social factors in illness and healthcare discussions on peer-to-peer forums*

A sub-field of medical education, called Narrative Medicine, uses illness narratives as resources for training of medical professionals. This rests on the premise that recognizing, interpreting, and being moved to action by the predicaments of patients improves the medical care being provided, and helps challenge purely biomedical accounts of illness. Rita Charon (2001), one of the founders of narrative medicine, for example, describes how her own practice of narrativizing her more difficult or troubling interactions with patients and then showing these stories to said patients led to faster disclosures of relevant details of people's medical histories (e.g. abuse) and to better relationships with her patients. This serves to illustrate that illness and health are not just questions of individual biology and physiology. There are always social and societal dimensions to illness and health, in how we experience them, express them, and how they are seen by others.

Coltman-Patel et al. (2022), for example, looked at how parents talk about vaccinations on the online parenting forum Mumsnet Talk. They were interested in particular in the role that conflict played in such discussions, because both the topic of vaccinations and a particular section of Mumsnet Talk called 'Am I being unreasonable' (henceforth, AIBU) are known to invite confrontation. As with some of the studies described in Chapter 7, the authors used corpus linguistic tools, specifically analyses of keywords, to get a sense of what was happening in their 6-million-word dataset. The 6-milion words were made up of 895 threads, all discussing vaccination-related issues within AIBU.

Coltman-Patel et al. (2022) found clear evidence that conflict was a key characteristic of vaccination discussions on AIBU when compared with vaccination discussions on other parts of Mumsnet Talk. The comparison revealed 323 keywords, which were then categorized into 15 groups based on semantic similarity. There were three groups of keywords that included a number of words indicative of some form of conflict: Communication (with keywords like 'apologise', 'offensive', 'patronising'), Negative evaluation (e.g. 'smug', 'vile'), and Insults as defined in Impoliteness theory (Culpeper, 2011), with keywords like 'cunt', 'idiot', 'twat'. This provided empirical linguistic evidence of the idea that AIBU was indeed more confrontational than the rest of Mumsnet Talk (at least when it came to vaccination discussions), which is something that had only been established on the basis of Mumsnet users' impressions recorded in post-hoc surveys and interviews. But another group of keywords, labelled People, revealed something particularly relevant in terms of social relationships around illness.

The largest group of keywords in the People group related to kinship (e.g. 'in-laws', 'mother', 'newborns'). The concordance lines of these keywords, reflected a major trend in vaccination discussions on AIBU: original posts (the posts that start a new thread) tended to outline a problematic or conflict situation in relation to vaccinations that hinged on various family members having differing attitudes to vaccinations, often in the context of a health or medical issue. In Example 8.4 the original poster describes how she has been repeatedly challenged by her partner's mother for not vaccinating her son, and asks for confirmation that her irritation at this perceived interference is justified:

EXAMPLE 8.4

> Had another delightful invasion from the in-laws today. Dp's [Dear partner's] Mum ended the visit by telling me how wrong I was not to get ds [dear son] (14 months) vaccinated. We've been through this many a time, just wish she'd respect and accept our decision. Am I right in thinking this is none of her bloody business? (15-Jan-11).

A similar social conflict is described in a pro-vaccination context in Example 8.5. Here the original poster describes being criticized by some family members for giving her child both recommended and optional vaccinations:

EXAMPLE 8.5

> I have opted to vaccinate my toddler against chicken pox and meningitis b (4 separate jabs) at quite a cost, but one I consider to be worth it. Certain members of my family have told me this is unfair to my child (to put her through trauma of extra injections) and un-necessary. They are implying I am some sort of cotton wool parent to do this and I need to relax a bit more. She is also about to have the flu vaccine (nasal spray), to which they rolled their eyes, even though it is recommended by NHS. Would other people think this way of me? (24-Oct-14)

These scenarios, which the authors argue are typical in the data, suggest that attitudes and decisions about (childhood) vaccinations are not just individual choices, but are rather intertwined with sometimes challenging kinship and social relationships. There is further evidence of this pattern in the group of keywords labelled as Insults. Coltman-Patel et al. (2022) found that the keywords in this group are often used to insult (and are therefore are examples of conventionalized impoliteness, Culpeper, 2011) specific people, and that these people are most frequently the family members that are described in the original posts, i.e. the family members at the heart of the offline conflict about vaccinations being described. This is a very clear example of the social context of healthcare that we outlined earlier, and it is important to be aware of this in debates around how to address vaccine hesitancy. If indecision or delays about vaccinations are not just caused by, for example, medical concerns, logistical challenges, misinformation or generally anti-science attitudes – factors that appear most frequently in the medical literature and which professionals are therefore prepared to address – but also by family pressure, peer group attitudes, and attempts to balance social, moral, and health concerns with maintaining close, personal relationships, then this aspect of people's social experience also needs to be considered and explored in consultations for example.

A different kind of social, and in this case also societal, factor is revealed by online discussions of post-natal depression (PND). This is a condition that is highly stigmatized in society and that new parents therefore find difficult to talk to healthcare professionals about (NHS, 2016). In fact, the UK's national charity for pregnancy, birth and early parenthood, NCT, reports that around 30% of PND cases do not get discussed with clinicians and are therefore not treated. Peer-to-peer online fora can provide an opportunity for people to speak more openly about their experiences, and help researchers (and healthcare professionals) learn more about the experience of the condition.

Kinloch and Jaworska (2020) conducted one such study using corpus linguistic analysis to look at the collocations (see Chapter 2) of the acronym 'PND' in discussions, also on the parenting site Mumsnet (among other datasets). Parenting websites can be really useful sources of data for health concerns around conception, pregnancy, birth and childhood. Kinloch and Jaworska found that in mothers' accounts (in this case it was predominantly mothers), PND collocates, i.e. frequently occurs together, with the terms 'severe', 'my', 'but', and 'cause' (among others), as in the examples below:

EXAMPLE 8.6

Along with a lot of other posters I've been there too, and PND was more severe than any of the other bouts of depression I have suffered from previously.

EXAMPLE 8.7

My PND was certainly caused/exacerbated by extreme sleep deprivation.

EXAMPLE 8.8

So yes – the pressure of bf [breastfeeding] can cause PND. It doesn't work the same for everyone.

EXAMPLE 8.9

PND is as much caused by the hormone changes as events around delivery although traumatic events can make you more susceptible to it

PND is sometimes dismissed by healthcare professionals, partly because it is without a clear-cut aetiology. The aetiological uncertainty leaves mothers with an explanatory burden trying to identify and locate the 'cause' of their symptoms often in external circumstances, e.g. lack of sleep, hormones, traumatic events (Example 8.7 and Example 8.9), highlighting that the actual experience varies from person to person (Example 8.7 and Example 8.8), while simultaneously signalling that their symptoms are legitimate and worthy of the PND label ('severe' in Example 8.6).

It appears that some mothers online are also ready to offer and accept alternative (as signalled by 'but' in Example 8.10), perhaps more established diagnoses such as stress, depression, and anxiety.

EXAMPLE 8.10

> The HV [health visitor] was concerned I may have PND, but I don't think I did, I think I was just exhausted & stressed.

The authors note that PND is a stigmatized condition (mothers often refer to 'hiding' it or 'admitting' they have it) because it contrasts too strongly with the ideals of (new) motherhood. In this social context, the external explanations (hormones, lack of sleep, etc.) and alternative diagnoses may serve to reduce the (self-)stigma associated with PND.

Similarly to Coltman-Patel et al.'s study, Kinloch and Jaworska demonstrate the importance of looking beyond the biomedical side of conditions such as PND, in order to be able recognize the unhelpful connections of PND with expectations of 'good' motherhood. This can help facilitate non-stigmatizing discussions with mothers both in public discourse and in healthcare consultations. Noting a similar pattern in a different online forum, Kantrowitz-Gordon (2013) suggested that healthcare providers need to find ways to make it safer for women to talk about postpartum depression.

The learning that can take place from exploring lived-experience accounts online is similar to what can be learnt from published memoirs and fictional accounts whether in the form of novels or multimedia. In fact, similar analyses can, of course, also be conducted on elicited data, such as focus groups discussions, interviews, or free-text responses to questionnaires. For example, Bullo (2020) conducted a metaphor analysis of descriptions of endometriosis pain collected via free-text responses to a questionnaire. Endometriosis – a painful condition where tissue similar to the lining of the womb grows in other places, such as the ovaries and fallopian tubes – is another stigmatized and marginalized condition that takes many years to diagnose, because women find it difficult to talk about and to get doctors to take them seriously. She found that women use elaborate metaphorical scenarios to convey the intensity of their pain and suggested that these might contrast with expected ways of describing pain or illnesses, thereby possibly leading to minimization, dismissal, or even misdiagnoses.

When content is elicited in some way, rather than collected from online forums, and the objective is to gather people's experiences and thoughts for the purposes of further linguistic analysis, then it is important that respondents or interviewees have as much space as possible to speak or write openly and freely, without much intervention from the researcher. A small number of very broad and open questions such as 'tell me about your experience of … ' tend to work best for this purpose (see also 'semi-structured interviews' in section 8.3.3 below and further guidance on interviews in Chapter 3).

Returning now to the kind of digital communication at the heart of this chapter, most online data has an interactive element. This sets it apart from other technologies for sharing experiences such as memoirs. We now turn to studies of this interactive nature of digital health communication.

8.3.2 Mutual support and community building in peer-to-peer forums

In addition to enabling a more holistic understanding of illness and healthcare experiences, online peer-to-peer fora dedicated to specific conditions or treatments are used because they can foster support and a sense of community among people who are going through similar things. In the introductory examples (Example 8.1–Example 8.3), you saw how an interesting linguistic feature of a single thread (the use of 'Mr' to refer to cancer) on an online forum dedicated to cancer can contribute to self-empowerment and community building. But the research team behind the project called 'Metaphor in End-of-Life Care' (Semino et al., 2018) was able to ask additional questions too. They had a 1.5-million-word corpus of online forum contributions by and interviews with patients, healthcare professionals, and family carers at their disposal. One of their main questions, in line with the name of the project, was: what kinds of metaphors are used by the different stakeholders and how? In this section, we focus on one part of their data, the online contributions by patients, and specifically on the Violence related metaphors that they found here.

Semino et al. (2018) conducted an initial qualitative analysis of a sample of their corpus identifying metaphors and assigning a source domain label to metaphorically used words. Metaphors were identified using the Metaphor Identification Procedure (Pragglejaz Group, 2007), which provides step-by-step instructions for how to decide whether a word is being used metaphorically or not. For a detailed discussion you need to refer to the original paper, but overall it is as follows: you start by reading the entire text to gain a general understanding of it. You then look at each word or 'lexical unit' (e.g. a compound verb) to establish what it means in the specific context (contextual meaning), such as 'battle' in 'my battle against cancer'. You then look up the same word in a dictionary, ideally a corpus-based one, to determine if it has a more 'basic' meaning as well. 'Basic meaning' here is a technical term denoting a meaning that is more concrete, related to bodily action, more precise, or historically older (such as 'a fight between two armies in a war' for 'battle'). If the word you are interested in does have a more basic meaning, and this contrasts with the contextual meaning but the latter can be understood in comparison with the former, then that word or lexical unit is used metaphorically.

Once a metaphor was identified, it was categorized according to the source domain or basic meaning of the word. For example, 'fighter', 'fight', and 'soldier' in Examples 8.11–8.13 were categorized as 'Violence' metaphors. Semino et al. (2018) then made use of the automatic semantic tagger 'USAS' built into the software Wmatrix (Rayson, 2009), as outlined in Chapter 7. They identified the USAS tags automatically assigned to all the metaphors they had manually categorized as a particular type, e.g. 'Violence'. Unsurprisingly, they found that many of the manually identified Violence metaphors like 'fighter', 'fight' and 'soldier' were categorized as 'G3 Warfare, defence and the army; weapons' by the automatic semantic tagger. The researchers then concordanced G3 (and other relevant USAS categories) to identify further metaphors.

Semino et al. (2018) found that many words in the 'Warfare, defence and the army; weapons' semantic category were indeed being used metaphorically in the patient data, i.e. were further examples of Violence metaphors. This was interesting because the metaphors they identified were very similar to so-called War metaphors that have often been criticized in the context of cancer and other illnesses (see Chapter 10), both in the media and scholarly work. Such critiques tend to point out that describing cancer as a war positions patient and illness as opponents, and implies that if someone does not recover then they are 'losing' the metaphorical battle. This places an unrealistic responsibility on cancer patients as they may be perceived, or perceive themselves, as not having fought hard enough. War metaphors have these kinds of implications, because, like all metaphors, they highlight some aspects of an experience while backgrounding others. This is known as the framing effect of metaphors (Entman, 1993). But some of the Violence metaphors that Semino et al. (2018) identified in the patient data had much more positive implications. The Violence metaphors, underlined in the examples below, for instance, were used interactionally, i.e. were directed at each other, rather than describing someone's personal experience:

EXAMPLE 8.11

You're such a <u>fighter</u> and so inspirational

EXAMPLE 8.12

keep up the good <u>fight</u>

EXAMPLE 8.13

<u>soldier</u> on everybody

These interactional uses of the Violence metaphor tended to suggest a determined and optimistic attitude, a sense of pride, enabling people to express praise and support for one another.

A small sub-set of Violence metaphors were also used humorously, with the forum participants fighting together against cancer (Example 8.14), and the healthcare system (Example 8.15). It turned out that these mainly occurred on the same humorous thread as the introductory 'Mr Crab/Cancer' examples:

EXAMPLE 8.14

> Cancer is the reason we are all here, so let's all <u>fight</u> that as an <u>army</u> together, <u>chaaaaaaaaaaaaarge</u>.

EXAMPLE 8.15

> It's got to be good results Valerie or they've made a mistake. Don't forget we have a formidable <u>fighting force</u> in our <u>rescue</u> team which now has two successful <u>missions</u> under their belts.

EXAMPLE 8.16

> as there has to be one as official <u>armourer</u> for warped I will put some balls of wool in the <u>armoury</u>

There were many of these examples on the Warped thread and Semino et al. (2018) showed that these were actually connected to each other. They formed part of extended metaphorical mini-narratives, or 'scenarios' (cf. Musolff, 2006) where the forum contributors were being collectively constructed as an army (Example 8.14), or members of a team who rescued their peers from hospital if they were kept there too long (Example 8.15). Cancer was the enemy (Example 8.14), and some contributors even had specific roles like that of armourer looking after weapons in the armoury (Example 8.16). This metaphor scenario tended to occur on the thread when contributors wrote about going for a check-up and being afraid of bad news or of having to stay in hospital Having to stay in hospital was seen as being held captive. Within the metaphor scenario, contributors position themselves as a collective army willing to physically fight for the person in hospital and even willing to break them free, should they be kept there.

By examining such Violence metaphors in detail, the researchers showed that it was not the source domain or vehicle of the metaphor that mattered (whether it was a War/Violence metaphor or a Journey metaphor, for example). When it came to framing effects, it was important *how* a metaphor was used and *by whom*: 'the framing effects of metaphors are a context- and usage-dependent phenomenon' (Semino et al, 2018: 3). They captured these nuances with the term 'empowerment'. Empowering uses of metaphor were those that represented the person with cancer in an agentive way, able to control or freely react to events for their own benefit, if they so wished, regardless of the source domain. The interactional and humorous Violence metaphors in the patient data tended to be empowering in this sense.

The activities described within the humorous metaphor scenarios are high-effort, high-impact actions where the contributors give themselves and each other a lot of agency. The contributors also express support and solidarity with the scenario, empathizing with each other's desire to not remain in hospital and providing a humorous distraction for each other in uncomfortable and anxiety-inducing situations offline. They effectively empower each other. Furthermore, the action of contributing to the online forum can itself be empowering: there is collaboration and collective effort in co-creating the metaphorical scenario. The resulting co-constructed scenario also functions in the same way as the Mr Cancer/Crab examples earlier. By knowing what this scenario is about and being able to contribute to it successfully people become part of the community.

Like with much other scholarly work, a lot of the research on online peer-to-peer health interactions tends to focus on Western, and global North contexts. That being said, there is evidence that such fora are used similarly in non-Western, global South contexts. As Kgatitswe (2012) suggests, for example, more and more people are turning to online peer support forums for their health needs in South Africa as well. She examines the use of these forums by women with breast cancer and shows that, although some of the affordances are different (e.g. platforms are often set up by patients rather than organizations and members are often friends and family members in real life, so they are less anonymous), they similarly help affected women find support, solidarity, and a sense of community.

In the next study, Stommel and Koole (2010) look at how interactional norms can have similar community building effects using a version of Conversation Analysis (CA) combined with Membership Categorization Analysis (MCA) (see Chapter 6 for the application of CA to in-person communication). This method allows them to look in detail at how group norms are communicated between participants and to new joiners. In fact, Stommel and Koole look at the ways in which specific linguistic behaviours that build a community can also function to *exclude* people on an online forum on eating disorders. They ask 'how do new members enter the forum and which expectations or implicit requirements are invoked in this process?'

Stommel and Koole (2010) note that newcomers to the eating disorder forum often present themselves in their first post via certain categories relevant to the group. Angela in Example 8.17 categorizes herself in terms of age and the eating disorder (ED) labels A (for anorexia) and B (for Bulimia) in the translation from German (NB: the original German is presented first, followed by the same text translated verbatim by the original authors):

EXAMPLE 8.17

1. *06.04.2005 15:57 From:* Angela *Subject:* Hallo, stell mich jetzt auch mal vor …
2. [...] Hi, ich bin [23–30], habe seit etwas über 8 Jahren ES, angefangen mit
3. MS, dann B★★, aber die Geschichten teilen wir ja leider hier fast alle … [...]

1. *06.04.2005 15:57 From:* Angela *Subject:* Hello, will also introduce myself …
2. *[…] Hi, I am [23–30], have had an ED for just over 8 years, began with*
3. *A, then B**, but unfortunately almost everybody here shares these stories … […]*

By declaring that these categories apply to her, Angela implicitly categorizes herself as ill and legitimizes her registration on the website and her contribution to the forum. As this is an interactional space, these legitimation strategies need to be acknowledged and affirmed by existing members in order for a new person to become part of the community. This is exactly what happens when Lucy responds to Angela in Example 8.18 with a warm welcome and by claiming the same membership categories for herself:

EXAMPLE 8.18

5. *07.04.2005 07:16 From:* Lucy *Subject:* Re: Hallo, stell mich jetzt auch mal vor …
6. Hallo Angela!!
7. Willkommen erstmal!!! *freu*
8. Ich erzähl mal von mir, okay? Ich bin [23–30] und hab seit etwa 14 Jahren B,
9. abwechselend mit MS. […]

5. *07.04.2005 07:16 From:* Lucy *Subject:* Re: Hello, will also introduce myself...
6. *Hello Angela!!*
7. *Firstly, welcome!!! *happy**
8. *I'll tell you something about me, okay? I'm [23–30] and have had B for about 14*
9. *years, alternating with A. […]*

The particular eating disorder forum in question is one that explicitly rejects so-called 'pro-anorexia', or anorexia glamourizing, attitudes, and considers anorexia, bulimia, and so on to be illnesses. Angela's self-categorization subscribed to these norms from the start and her entry into the community was smooth. Becoming part of the same community with a different attitude to these conditions is considerably more difficult, as Example 8.19 and Example 8.20 show:

EXAMPLE 8.19

1. *02.04.2005 10:18 From:* Doreen *Subject:* ziemlich unsicher
2. Hallo mal an alle! ich bin mir nicht wirklich sicher ob ich hier richtig bin, mir hat
3. ne freundin den Rat gegeben mal hier zu schreiben,
4. es is die einzige die mich je hätte zu sowas bringen können!
5. Gut um es auf den Punkt zu bringen,
6. ich bin jetzt seit einem jahr ["magersuchtsverherrlichend"]
7. aber ich bin mir nicht sicher ob das richtig ist, und ob ich wirklich krank bin,

8.   oder nur krank sein will, das weiß ich einfach nicht,

9.   ich persönlich seh es einfach nicht ein, wenn jemand sagt,

10. dass ich krank bin oder dass ich ein problem hab!!

1.   *02.04.2005 10:18 From:* Doreen *Subject:* quite unsure

2.   *Hi everyone! I'm not really sure if I'm in the right place,*

3.   *a friend advised me to write here,*

4.   *she is the only person that could have made me do something like this!*

5.   *Good, to get to the point,*

6.   *I've been ['glamorizing anorexia'] for one year,*

7.   *but I'm not sure if that's right, and whether I'm really ill,*

8.   *or only want to be ill, I simply don't know,*

9.   *personally I simply don't see it when someone says*

10. *I'm ill or that I've got a problem!!*

In Example 8.19 Doreen explicitly questions whether she could belong to the category of 'ill', and instead claims the category of 'anorexia glamourizing' for herself, albeit also ambivalently. In this way, she does not unequivocally subscribe to the category norms of the group, but also not to the counter categories. The responses, in multiple ways, are both friendly and welcoming, but also only allow a partial entry into the community. Just before Example 8.20, Paula welcomes Doreen warmly (acceptance into the group), but also tries to encourage Doreen towards accepting the illness category by pointing out that an attachment to being underweight is 'not healthy'. She also says the following:

EXAMPLE 8.20

1.   *02.04.2005 16:30 From:* Paula *Subject:* Re: ziemlich unsicher

2.   Hier kann man nicht versagen!

3.   Aber lass die Finger von [den krankheitsverrlichenden Seiten],

4.   das ist doch der totale Wahnsin …

1.   *02.04.2005 16:30 From:* Paula *Subject:* Re: quite unsure

2.   *It's not possible to fail here!*

3.   *But keep away from the [glamorizing illness sites],*

4.   *That's just total madness …*

In line 2, Paula again accepts Doreen into the community, by rejecting the possibility of failing as a member, but also provides a directive for what Doreen needs to still do to gain full access to the community in line 3. With this analysis (more extensive in the original), Stommel and Koole (2010) show that self-categorization in interaction can and does contribute to building communities online, but it can also make it difficult for new contributors to become part of the same community. If someone is not able or willing to display the right attitude or identity, they risk being excluded, even if only partially.

Identity and stance are of course not just relevant for interactional online data, and a different reason for exploring how people categorize, describe, and present themselves in their lived-experience accounts online is to understand what role online environments play in their illness experience and what implications this might have for more public communication strategies about illness. This is the subject of the next section in relation to social media.

8.3.3 Identities, expertise, and authenticity in lived-experience narratives on social media

Koteyko and Hunt (2016) explored identity construction via a four-month lon-gitudinal online observation of 20 Facebook accounts belonging to people with type 1 and type 2 diabetes. Diabetes is a chronic condition which can impact how people see themselves and how others see them, so identity is particularly rel-evant here. Koteyko and Hunt complemented their observation with subsequent semi-structured interviews, a method that relies on asking often broad ques-tions within a thematic framework, but without a fixed order or phrasing. Their research questions include: what are the linguistic and semiotic resources used by people with diabetes to manage and organize their identities on Facebook? How is their use of the site's architectural affordances involved in such identity construction? What can such identity performances tell us about the implications of social networking site use for narrating illness experiences?

Along with many studies of identity using sociolinguistic and discourse approaches, Koteyko and Hunt draw on the post-structuralist view on identity, which sees identity as constructed (rather than reflected) in discourse, and as emergent (Bucholtz & Hall, 2005). This is a framework we highlight in Chapters 1 and 6 as well, and within it, the following can all contribute to the emergence of identity: 'an explicit mention of identity categories and labels, evaluative ori-entations to ongoing talk as well as interactive footings, and the use of linguis-tic phenomena that have ideological associations' (Bucholtz & Hall, 2005: 594) (2016: 61).

Social media sites like Facebook are different from peer support forums as dis-cussed in previous sections because, generally speaking, they are less anonymous and more anchored to non-digital life. They are also spaces with a high degree of 'context collapse' (Marwick & boyd, 2011), where individuals are broadcasting to multiple different audience groups simultaneously (work colleagues, family, childhood friends from school, etc.), rather than directly writing to like-minded others within a closed group. These distinctions all have a bearing on identity construction.

Koteyko and Hunt (2016) adopted a discourse-oriented ethnography design for their study, which consisted of online participant observation and detailed text analysis. Ethnography generally refers to the study of people and cultural phenomena, including language, 'from within', i.e. from the point of view of the person or phenomenon being studied. This type of analysis requires that the researcher enter the participants' life-world (in this case, their digital world) to examine their situated use of social media and discourse, in addition to observable patterns of language. In other words, there is a focus not just on the end product (the texts and images created and shared), but also on the behaviours, processes, and practices around it. This type of observation allows us to begin to understand what role these interactions play in the lives and identity construction of people, in this case, with diabetes. The authors focused specifically on what the participants post, how they do it, i.e. what modes (visual, verbal, architectural affordances of the site, etc.) they use, and what meanings are created. It is important to note that this type of research is only ethical if individual consent is obtained from participants (see Chapter 3), and this is exactly what Koteyko and Hunt did.

The authors found that participants used the platform to construct personal expertise in relation to diabetes management; to display their own integration into wider diabetes-related networks; to report on mundane aspects of diabetes self-management; to negotiate professional and cultural expectations of diabetes self-management in a playful manner.

The construction or display of expertise has been noted in numerous studies of computer-mediated interaction around health (including Stommel & Koole, 2010 above) and relates to the need to support or legitimize any advice or suggestions among peers with some reference to one's source of expertise. This can be done via explicit statements such as 'I've had T1 for 49 yrs and never had any support as a teen!' to accompany advice on letting a teenage child learn to manage their own diabetes. But the ethnographic and longitudinal methodology that Koteyko and Hunt (2016) employed also allowed them to demonstrate how this type of expertise can be signalled more subtly over a longer period of time. They noted that many participants used the affordances of Facebook to construct themselves as experts in diabetes by regularly 'liking' informational posts published on the pages of diabetes organizations and republishing or 'sharing' these posts to their networks, together with their own (simple) evaluative commentary, e.g. commenting 'The way forward for blood testing' on an article detailing a new type of glucose monitoring system. In this way they positioned themselves, not just as experts by experience, but also as translators of recent developments in the medical field of diabetes and diabetes management. The use of first person pronouns, medical terminology, and factual content were typical of this activity, but the authors were able to show how the practices afforded by Facebook's infrastructure also played an important role and, in fact, provided participants with alternative ways of performing their expert-by-experience identity.

Facebook enabled participants not just to construct themselves as (different types of) experts by experience, but also to bring together their multiple identities, e.g. as a self-managing diabetic, a fun person, a 'normal' person. This bringing together of multiple identities was facilitated by the typical 'context collapse' feature of social media. Participants in Koteyko and Hunt's study exploited the

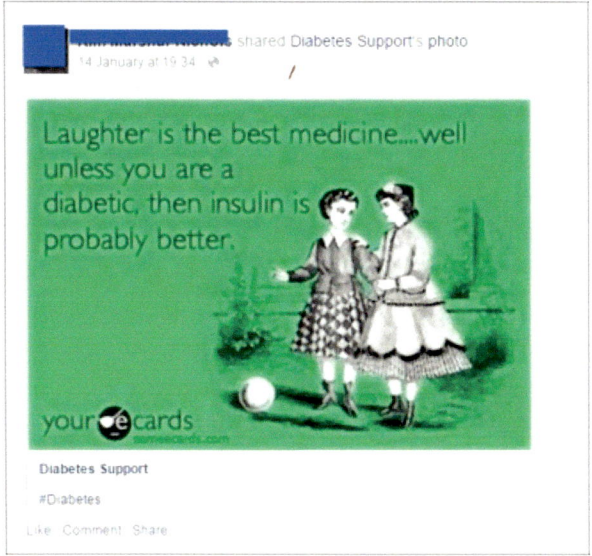

FIGURE 8.1   Humorous diabetes meme from Koteyko and Hunt (2016)

collapsed context of Facebook to index that their identities do not just consist of being diabetic. For example, one participant took part in a Facebook 'challenge' to share 'things you may not know about me'. The participant provided a long list of recreational and spiritual activities and only briefly referred to having diabetes. Another participant posted humorous diabetes-related memes (such as Figure 8.1) to their own timeline (as opposed to a diabetes specific group) to share more widely that they are living with diabetes while also signalling a (relatively) light-hearted approach to the condition and its seriousness. In this way they were able to maintain a cohesive profile while also signalling multiple and mutable identities.

As indicated in Koteyko and Hunt's study, people's experiences of illness are captured and shared in increasingly multimodal ways. People with different illnesses don't just use social networking sites or write blogs, but also produce and share videos of themselves narrating their experiences. The fact that the people in these videos have direct experience of the illness plays a large part in the attention they receive. One study exploring what makes video-based illness narratives engaging is Chou et al.'s (2011) exploration of cancer narratives on YouTube.

Chou et al. (2011) collected 35 YouTube stories posted by cancer survivors, transcribed them for analysis, and conducted a language-based narrative analysis to understand how 'authentic' illness experiences are structured in this medium (see Chapter 12 on the importance of authenticity in medical contexts). In linguistic studies the structure of narratives is often described with reference to Labov and Waletzky's (1967) classic study on the structure of oral narratives (even when written narratives are concerned). In their study, Labov and Waletzky recorded the stories told when they asked people whether they had ever been in danger of dying. As outlined in Labov (1972), the 'narratives of personal experience' produced in response to this question were told in remarkably similar ways. They tended to include the following five main elements:

- Abstract: an indication that the speaker has a story to tell and/or a brief summary;
- Orientation: a description of the setting, including time, place, people, situation;
- Evaluation: devices that indicate the point of the story, that is, why it is worth telling. These tend to be peppered throughout the narrative;
- Complicating action: a series of clauses that present the events that are the core of the story;
- Resolution: an indication of the final event;
- Coda: an indication that the story is finished and potentially some general observations on the effects of the event on the narrator.

Chou et al. (2011) used this classic structure of narratives to analyze the YouTube cancer stories and understand whether and how *the way in which* these authentic stories are told can be harnessed to improve communications promoting desirable health behaviours.

Firstly, they discovered that, after a brief abstract, all videos in their dataset established themselves as diagnostic narratives in the orientation phase. The stories centred around the person's experience of the diagnosis and made little, and mostly impersonal, reference to the medical professionals who delivered the diagnosis. The diagnosis in question was invariably presented as unexpected and highly memorable through the use of specific dates and descriptions of the mundane activities that were ongoing at the time of diagnosis:

EXAMPLE 8.21

> For me life basically consists of basketball, football, soccer, and video games. But in May of 2006 I was diagnosed with cancer in my left arm.

Dramatic tension was further increased through the use of directly reported speech and explicit evaluation throughout the story:

EXAMPLE 8.22

> Um, but I said, I think I felt something in the shower. He said, Well you're young, I'm sure it's nothing, but let me check it out anyway.

EXAMPLE 8.23

> You find yourself just in a surreal place like this can't really be happening to me, it was a mistake.

Direct speech is known to pull the audience into the here-and-now of the narrative and increase the immediacy of the narrated events in speech (Tannen, 2005; see also Chapter 5 for its role in published novels and memoirs), while Labovian evaluation helps make explicit the point and impact of the story. These features serve to increase the emotional engagement of audiences, contributing to the effectiveness of these videos as communication tools.

Another relevant feature of these YouTube narratives was the occasional switch from first-person 'I' narration to the use of the generic second person pronoun 'you', in bold in the example below:

EXAMPLE 8.24

> I'm doing pretty good today and I'm breaking it down. But at the time **you**'re overwhelmed by this news. It's just too much! **You** think **you**'re dying you know, according to them. And the way **you** cough, I felt like it.

Chou et al. (2011) argue that, on the one hand, this signals a sense of lack of control over the events on the speaker's part. This is particularly evident in Example 5.23 in combination with 'find yourself'. On the other hand, the use of the generic 'you' also served to increase engagement with the audience, both because 'you' always carries the hint of direct address and because it suggests that the experiences and reactions being described are not unique to the speaker. The implication is that anyone in the same position would feel the same way.

Overall, Chou et al. (2011) aimed to better understand what the common linguistic elements of YouTube cancer narratives are and how these might help to reach and engage audiences. This has very real implications for the health of those watching the videos, since engagement with survivors' narratives has been shown to lead to desirable health behaviours, such as increased mammography uptake among African American women in the US (Kreuter et al., 2008). Chou et al. (2011) summarize that cancer communication programmes using narratives should emulate the narrative structure and associated linguistic features of these YouTube videos to increase the likelihood of resonating with their intended audiences. In line with the philosophy of Narrative Medicine they too suggest that clinicians in direct interaction with patients might also benefit from listening to such stories. They might understand patients' perspectives better and therefore be able to offer more appropriate support.

Although the focus of this chapter was interactions between and lived-experience accounts by people who have health concerns, it is of course possible and indeed worthwhile to also study such texts when they are produced by healthcare practitioners and clinicians. Charon's work, mentioned earlier, already alluded to this, but it is certainly not just the lived-experience of physicians that is of interest. Some of the data in the project that Semino et al. (2018) describe comes from interactions between different healthcare practitioners and it is revealing that they too find support and solidarity online, even if they generally write less, and less freely, in the online public domain.

8.4 Concluding remarks

Lived-experience accounts online represent rich sources of information and data when it comes to illness and health. They can help us understand the social and societal, as well as subjective and personal, aspects of illness and healthcare. They can reveal insights about group dynamics and self-presentation in the context of illness. And they can point towards people's use of technologies to help them cope in different ways.

Digital data tends to come in large quantities so corpus methods are often used for linguistic analysis. However, other, more manually intensive methods such as narrative analysis and digital ethnography are equally appropriate. And indeed, similar analyses to those outlined in this chapter can be performed on lived-experience accounts elicited in interviews or free-text responses to surveys.

Further readings

Baker, P. (2006). *Using corpora in discourse analysis*. Continuum.

Bucholtz, M., & Hall, K. (2005). Identity and interaction: A sociocultural linguistic approach. *Discourse Studies*, 7(4–5), 585–614.

De Fina, A., & Georgakopoulou, A. (2015). *The handbook of narrative analysis*. Wiley.

Georgakopoulou, A., & Spilioti, T. (Eds.). (2015). *The Routledge handbook of language and digital communication*. Routledge. Especially chapters 4, 20, and 21.

References

Bucholtz, M., & Hall, K. (2005). Identity and interaction: A sociocultural linguistic approach. *Discourse Studies*, 7(4–5), 585–614.

Bullo, S. (2020). "I feel like I'm being stabbed by a thousand tiny men": The challenges of communicating endometriosis pain. *Health*, 24(5), 476–492.

Cepeda, M. S., Chapman, C. R., Miranda, N., Sanchez, R., Rodriguez, C. H., Restrepo, A. E., Ferrer, L. M., Linares, R. A., & Carr, D. B. (2008, June). Emotional disclosure through patient narrative may improve pain and well-being: Results of a randomized controlled trial in patients with cancer pain. *Journal of Pain and Symptom Management*, 35(6), 623–631.

Charon, R. (2001). Narrative medicine: Form, function, and ethics. *Annals of Internal Medicine*, 134(1), 83–87.

Chou, W.-Y. S., Hunt, Y., Folkers, A., & Augustson, E. (2011). Cancer survivorship in the age of YouTube and social media: A narrative analysis. *Journal of Medical Internet Research*, *13*(1), 108–116.

Coates, J. (2007). Talk in a play frame: More on laughter and intimacy. *Journal of Pragmatics*, *39*(1), 29–49.

Coltman-Patel, T., Dance, W., Demjén, Z., Gatherer, D., Hardaker, C., & Semino, E. (2022). 'Am I being unreasonable to vaccinate my kids against my ex's wishes?' – A corpus linguistic exploration of conflict in vaccination discussions on Mumsnet Talk's AIBU forum. *Discourse, Context, and Media*, *48*, 100624.

Culpeper, J. (2011). *Impoliteness. Using language to cause offence.* Cambridge University Press.

Demjén, Z. (2016). Laughing at cancer: Humour, empowerment, solidarity and coping online. *Journal of Pragmatics*, *101*, 18–30.

Entman, R. M. (1993). Framing: Toward clarification of a fractured paradigm. *Journal of Communication*, *43*(4), 51–58.

Galegher, J., Sproull, L., & Kiesler, S. (1998). Legitimacy, authority and community in electronic support groups. *Written Communication*, *15*(4), 493–530.

Kantrowitz-Gordon, I. (2013, December). Internet confessions of postpartum depression. *Issues in Mental Health Nursing*, *34*(12), 874–882.

Kgatitswe, L. B. (2012). "We're living in an era of facebook and blogs. It's a familiar and comfortable space": Exploring the use of virtual support groups by women diagnosed with breast cancer. Unpublished Master Research Report. University of Witwatersrand. Retrieved from https://core.ac.uk/download/pdf/39670409.pdf

Kinloch, K., & Jaworska, S. (2020). Using a comparative corpus-assisted approach to study health and illness discourses across domains: The case of postnatal depression (PND) in lay, medical and media texts. In Z. Demjén (Ed.), *Applying linguistics in illness and healthcare contexts*. Bloomsbury.

Koteyko, N., & Hunt, D. (2016). Performing health identities on social media: An online observation of Facebook profiles. *Discourse, Context and Media*, *12*, 59–67.

Kreuter, M. W., Buskirk, T. D., Holmes, K., Clark, E. M., Robinson, L., Si, X., Erwin, D., Philipneri, A., Cohen, E., & Mathews, K. (2008). What makes cancer survivor stories work? An empirical study among African American women. *Journal of Cancer Survivorship*, *2*(1), 33–44.

Labov, W. (1972). *Language in the inner city. Studies in the Black English vernacular/William Labov*. University of Pennsylvania Press.

Labov, W., & Waletzky, J. (1967 [1997]). Narrative analysis. In J. Helm (Ed.), *Essays on the verbal and visual arts* (pp. 12–44). University of Washington Press. Reprinted in *Journal of Narrative and Life History*, *7*(1–4), 3–38.

Marwick, A. E., & Boyd, D. (2011). I tweet honestly, I tweet passionately: Twitter users, context collapse, and the imagined audience. *New Media and Society*, *13*(1), 114–133.

Musolff, A. (2006). Metaphor scenarios in public discourse. *Metaphor and Symbol*, *21*(1), 23–38.

NHS. (2016). Postnatal depression. Retrieved December 21, 2017, from http://www.nhs.uk/Conditions/Postnataldepression/Pages/Introduction.aspx

Patsos, M. (2001). The Internet and medicine: Building a community for patients with rare diseases. *JAMA*, *285*(6), 805. https://doi.org/10.1001/jama.285.6.805-JMS0214-2-1

Pragglejaz Group. (2007). MIP: A method for identifying metaphorically used words in discourse. *Metaphor and Symbol*, *22*(1), 1–39.

Rayson, P. (2009). Wmatrix: A web-based corpus processing environment. Computing Department, Lancaster University. http://ucrel.lancs.ac.uk/wmatrix/

Semino, E., Demjén, Z., Hardie, A., Payne, S., & Rayson, P. (2018). *Metaphor, cancer, and the end of life: A corpus-based study*. Routledge.

Stommel, W., & Koole, T. (2010). The online support group as a community: A micro-analysis of the interaction with a new member. *Discourse Studies, 12*(3), 357–378.

Tannen, D. (2005). *Conversational style: Analyzing talk among friends*. Oxford University Press.

Thurnherr, F., Rudolf von Rohr, M., & Locher, M. (2016). The functions of narrative passages in three written online health contexts. *Open Linguistics, 2*(1). https://doi.org/10.1515/opli-2016-0024

PART III

Learning from research in language and health: Case studies

9

MEDICAL ADVERTISING AND MEDICALIZATION

A multimodal critical discourse analysis

9.1 Introduction and rationale

This book has presented a range of approaches to understanding health and healthcare which highlight people's lived experiences, and societal discourses and ideologies, all of which are helpful to address through linguistic methods. But how might you study something as huge as societal 'discourses' or 'ideologies' around health within a small scale, single study, of the type you might plan yourself for a project or dissertation?

This particular case study showcases Kevin Harvey's study 'Medicalisation, pharmaceutical promotion and the Internet: a critical multimodal discourse analysis of hair loss websites' (2013) which addresses the complex social phenomenon of 'medicalization', a term outlined further below, through the lens of eight websites, all of which advertise remedies for hair loss. This demonstrates how a very large topic in medical sociology can be approached and evidenced through close linguistic analysis of a particular real-life instance of that phenomenon. The study employed multimodal critical discourse analysis (MCDA), an approach also discussed in Chapter 4. Using linguistic methods in this way to empirically test claims from other disciplines means you can identify a general area of interest but then approach it through a close and systematic analysis of a manageable dataset, within a single study (see also Chapter 11). In fact, linking the 'macro' aspects of sociocultural practice to the 'micro' features of particular texts like this is very much an objective of Critical Discourse Analysis (Fairclough, 1992: 9). While you might not opt to use exactly the same topic as Harvey (2013) within your own project, we hope that it sparks some ideas around how to narrow down a research focus and dataset from an initial area of interest, draw on multimodal aspects of texts as part of your analysis and conduct high quality and systematic analyses of wider 'discourses', evidenced within your texts.

DOI: 10.4324/9781003020417-12

9.1.1 Key literature – Medicalization

Harvey (2013) collects a dataset of hair loss remedy websites to critically examine how they reconfigure what are sometimes considered natural processes of ageing into medical conditions that require treatment – demonstrating a wider sociocultural phenomenon of 'medicalization'. There is a variety of literature in medical sociology that is helpful to draw on in understanding medicalization. Harvey (2013) cites the seminal work of Conrad (1992) to define medicalization as the process by which aspects of everyday life become, 'defined and treated as medical problems, usually in terms of illnesses or disorders' (Conrad, 1992: 209). Conrad (2007) argues that this has increased over the past few decades and we might suggest it has increased further still since Conrad's defining work. More recently, Thomas (2021) similarly defined medicalization as the ways in which 'a growing array of conditions and experiences of human life become defined, understood, and managed through medical and medically-related expertise' (23). She highlights how this 'has been driven not only by the work of medical professionals, but increasingly by pharmaceutical companies and consumers' (2007: 23), through exactly the types of commercial, consumer-oriented websites that Harvey (2013) examines. Scholars highlight both the benefits and problems that come from this increasing medicalization of society. Harvey (2013) for example, while he does himself take a critical approach to the commercial promotion of hair loss remedies, highlights the work of scholars who have also argued for the social benefits of increasing medicalization, such as the prevention of underdiagnosis of serious disease (Bonaccorso & Sturchio, 2002) and encouraging greater access to clinical care (Ebrahim, 2002). However, by and large the concept of 'medicalization' has been used to critically examine structures of medical power in relation to lay persons. Thomas (2021) highlights how medicalization 'can shape, and be shaped by, dominant power structures and inequalities' and that this has implications 'for healthcare and treatment accessibility, associated cultures of working practice, and societal norms, values and expectations' (30). This is particularly the case for the commercial factors driving medicalization, including the market interests in promoting pharmaceutical remedies such as the hair loss remedies discussed here (Conrad, 2005, Mintzes, 2002; Brennan et al., 2009; Moynihan et al., 2002).

9.2 Methods and data

The concerns around medicalization outlined above, particularly how social processes are shaped by but also work to reinforce power structures, map well with the core concerns of Critical Discourse Analysis, as noted in Chapters 2 and 4. While there has been a good deal of discussion of pharmaceutical marketization within medical sociology, Harvey identifies a research gap in terms of the lack of attention to the marketing texts themselves, which work to promote pharmaceutical remedies to consumers through a variety of visual and textual strategies. He makes the case that the approaches of social semiotics and multimodal critical discourse analysis (MCDA) can provide a valuable methodology for gaining a detailed understanding of how marketing texts discursively enact this process of medicalization. MCDA is particularly useful for looking at the integrated use of visual features alongside the textual, an approach similarly adopted by Koteyko and Nerlich (2007) in analyzing pro-biotic advertising sites. Harvey employs the same approach to answer the following questions around hair loss remedy websites:

Discourse design
- Representations: what social actors and processes are depicted in the websites? How are these social actors represented in visual images and language?
- Negotiating identities and relations: what types of social relations are constructed (both in language and image) between the represented participants in the websites and readers/viewers? Further, what attitudes do the text and images convey to readers/viewers?

Discourse audience and reception
- How are readers/viewers of the websites positioned? Are they, for example, constructed as informed consumers or non-experts in need of scientific, medical advice?

Discourse as sociocultural practice
- What insights do the combined use of visual images and language reveal about the underlying ideologies of the websites, in particular their formulation of and responses to lifestyle problems such as hair loss?

(Harvey, 2013: 696)

9.2.1 Data selection

Once you have identified a particular phenomenon of interest, such as 'medicalization', how do you go about researching this? As outlined for this study, Harvey identified a particular realization of this phenomenon – hair loss remedies – and a source of data that was likely to demonstrate an instance of this – online adverts and marketing texts. You could equally choose a different instance, such as media representations of particular health conditions that contribute to medicalization. So, how do you go about establishing your criteria and selecting a collection of texts to analyze? In CDA, texts are often selected which are 'typical' of the phenomenon in question. Online advertising of hair loss remedies was a fruitful source for Harvey to turn to in this study, since, as Harvey highlights, the Internet has become a key conduit through which to market medicines to people in their day-to-day lives (Fox & Ward, 2008) and a medium through which many consumers seek out information on hair loss (Lovett, 2002). The same is likely to be true of many other conditions targeted by the pharmaceutical industries too and you may want to consider new areas in which marketing (online or otherwise) has become prominent. One of the difficulties Harvey faced was in fact the very large amount of potential data available online. As he states, a Google search using terms related to hair loss yielded hundreds of thousands of results, e.g.; 'hair loss' (114,000,000), 'baldness' (13,700,000), and 'Propecia' (65,600,000). Many studies drawing on Internet data face this dilemma of how to select a manageable research dataset from the vast amount of material that is readily available, an issue also discussed in Chapters 7 and 11. Harvey ultimately opted to select websites that appeared at the top of search engine results, with the rationale that these would be the most likely for consumers and information seekers to access.

This is not the only possible approach – in a similar study looking at the marketing of probiotics online, Koteyko and Nerlich (2007) opt to select websites on the basis of the most prominent commercial companies in this area, selecting four yoghurt making companies who had been listed as market leaders and four producers of supplements containing probiotics, who were featured in UK media coverage that they analyzed separately (Nerlich & Koteyko, 2008). Depending on the objectives of your study, there are a variety of approaches that can be used for selecting Internet data, such as identifying sites that have evidence of receiving the greatest amount of Internet traffic or websites published between certain dates. Bear in mind that if you are selecting sites on the basis of those which appear 'highest' in search results, these *intentionally* vary within search engine results according to geographical location, personal search histories and algorithm variations. The top results you gain might not therefore be the same in all contexts and you will need to acknowledge this potential limitation. Overall, it is important to be able to select data according to some kind of principle, justifying how you included (and excluded) material, keeping in mind that it is not sufficient to select websites on the basis that they simply provide the most interesting or easily analyzable data.

9.2.2 Semiotics and Multimodal Critical Discourse Analysis

The images and visual design of the websites Harvey selected were likely to be important to the meanings of the texts, therefore requiring an analytic approach that could incorporate these elements. Multimodality and Critical Discourse Analysis were introduced in Chapter 4 and the latter was defined as a 'theoretical perspective on language and more generally semiosis (including visual language, body language, and so on) […] Which gives rise to ways of analyzing language or semiosis within broader analyses of the social process' (Fairclough, 2001: 121). It is a useful approach for looking closely at how texts, which are viewed as a type of social practice, reflect but also construct or reinforce wider discourses and ideologies in society. Since this definition includes visual language, Chapter 4 (and Chapter 5) also introduced ideas on 'multimodality', i.e. that texts communicate meaning through multiple modes. The field of Critical Discourse Analysis in particular has argued for the importance of incorporating these multimodal features, such as layout and visual design, into an understanding of text, as well as the lexical features, since these other 'semiotic modes' also encode representations of power and ideology. Building on Halliday's (2013) systemic functional grammar, which has always been widely used in CDA, MCDA has developed systematic frameworks for analyzing visual design from a similar perspective. Harvey (2013) draws particularly on Kress and van Leeuwen's grammar of visual design (2020), which provides a framework for classifying how images encode representations of the external world or internal experience. For example, Kress and van Leeuwen (2020) distinguish images in terms of the direction of gaze, with a fundamental difference in the way a 'relationship' is created with the viewer depending on whether the represented participants look directly into the viewer's eyes – 'demand' images – or are the objects of the viewer's scrutiny – 'offer' images. This framework for considering agency and representation, between the participants represented and the viewer, fits with the aims of Critical Discourse Analysis in understanding the power relationships and ideologies encoded.

9.3 Results and discussion

From his analysis, Harvey identifies four discursive strategies across the eight websites used to represent male hair loss and its treatment. These are:

1. Representing the balding man as type and outcast;
2. Promoting the attractiveness and self-assurance of the hirsute man;
3. Situating male hair loss in a scientific discourse;
4. Encouraging consumers to self-evaluate their hair loss.

(Harvey, 2013: 696)

He structures his results through four sections, each elaborating on these four discourses in turn. Structuring the presentation of your results in this way, in terms of particular themes or discourses, provides a useful means of synthesizing your findings from across different data, rather than having to present an analysis of each website in turn.

9.3.1 Representing the balding man as type and outcast

In terms of this first discourse, Harvey (2013) identified two key configurations through which men were depicted in the visual imagery of the websites. The first was men depicted as lone figures in some remote setting, illustrated in Figure 9.1, where an image of a man is looking out to sea, prominently displayed on one of the websites Harvey analyzed. A slogan 'save the hair' appears in a large font, with a strapline marketing the pharmaceutical product just below it; 'with PROPECIA, 9 out of 10 men had visible results'. Employing Kress and

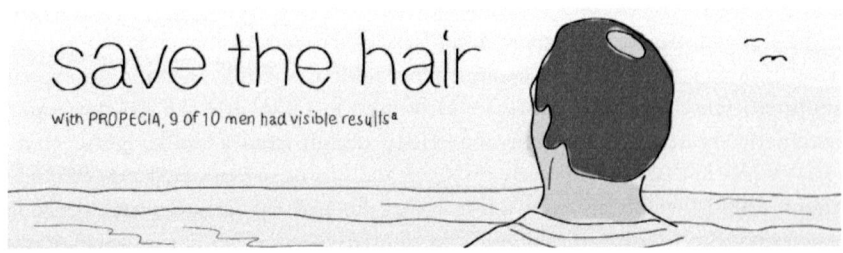

FIGURE 9.1 Image of lone man on beach (Propecia.com)

van Leeuwen's framework, Harvey identifies this image of a man, with his gaze turned away, as an 'offer' image, that is, an image in which the represented participants are offered 'to the viewer as items of information, objects of contemplation' (Kress & van Leeuwen, 2020: 119). Here, Harvey suggests that the balding man is represented as an impersonal 'other' with whom audiences are not invited to connect. With few other physical features and no 'actions' presented in the image, Harvey suggests that the viewer is also encouraged to see the man *in terms of* his baldness, backgrounding any other characteristic.

In MCDA, it is useful to show examples of the images analyzed as part of your written analysis, just as you would in giving extracts from written texts. It can also be helpful to reproduce the images you analyze more extensively as part of an appendix, although you should of course check the guidelines for the particular piece of work you are producing. However, Harvey faced a particular difficulty in publishing his analysis of the visual aspects of these websites, where issues of copyright were encountered in reproducing the images, (see Chapter 3). To address this difficulty, Harvey commissioned an artist to create illustrations of the original images, allowing him to show sufficient visual information to demonstrate his multimodal analysis with Kress and van Leeuwen's (2020) framework. Where you are producing a report as part of a module assessment, you may well be able to use the original images within 'fair use' policies for education and so are unlikely to encounter copyright restrictions. Where you are seeking to produce a piece of work that you would later like to publish though, as can be the case for some Master's dissertations and PhDs, you may need to consider issues of copyright quite carefully, to ensure that the analysis you conduct can be used.

Harvey is careful to integrate analysis of the image with the textual elements of this composition. The imperative 'save the hair' overlaid on the image is not a peripheral element but an essential part of the design, 'both compositionally and semantically [...] positioned as it is within the confines of the image itself and contributing to its interactive meaning' (Harvey, 2013: 698). In this case, Harvey (2013) suggests that the imperative 'save the hair' acts almost as a warning to those viewing the website and very directly urges the audience to act in order to stop hair falling out. Harvey's study provides a good example of the value in considering these elements together in MCDA approaches.

9.3.2 Promoting the attractiveness and self-assurance of the hirsute man

This first discourse contrasts starkly with the compositions identified as part of the second key discourse in Harvey's list of four, *Promoting the attractiveness and self-assurance of the hirsute man*. For this discourse, images usually depicted men with full heads of hair looking straight towards the camera, in what Kress and van Leeuwen (2020) define as 'demand' images, actively inviting some kind of relationship with the viewer. For example, in Figure 9.2, from another hair loss remedy website, an 'ideal' man with full hair is shown in close up. While some of the images of balding men were also shown in close up, Harvey (2013) argues that the difference in the direction of gaze from the first image (in Figure 9.2, directly towards the viewer) encourages the viewer to engage or identify with the participant, and invites them to connect having a full head of hair with confidence and contentment.

Again, the image is combined with textual elements, promoting the product Propecia as a hair loss 'treatment that works', making the important connection between this representation of the 'ideal' man and the pharmaceutical route to achieving this. An image of the product is given in the bottom right-hand corner that does itself have the stark gendered claim 'For Men Only' on the packaging, with Harvey highlighting how the websites construct hair loss as a threat to a man's masculinity.

You should keep in mind of course that readers are not simply passive entities and that they may vary in how they interpret these images. Harvey highlights that some website users may not consciously register the values and social relations encoded in the discourses or might resist or contest these. Nevertheless, it is possible to analyze these choices as having an underlying ideology in the way they represent baldness and masculinity.

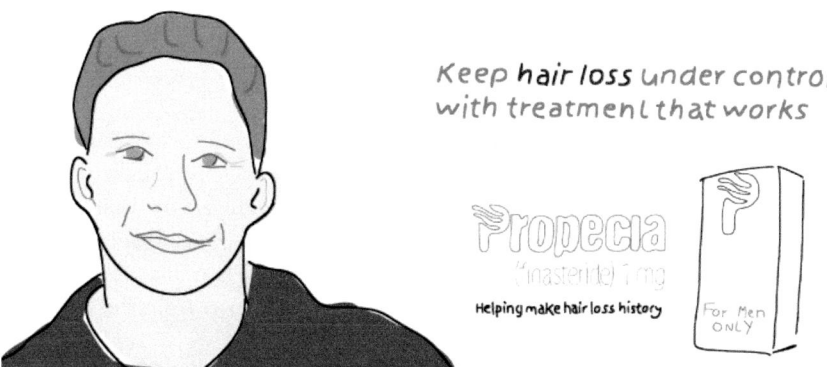

FIGURE 9.2   Image of smiling man (Propeciaonline)

9.3.3 Situating male hair loss in a scientific discourse

For discourse 3, Harvey highlights how some elements in the texts are embedded in a wider social discourse or perhaps 'genre' of scientific language. Here the website texts draw on social norms and values around the use of technical language and evidence for medical treatments for baldness, to 'represent this as an indisputably scientific problem' (p. 706). Harvey also highlights how this technical, biological discourse is combined with more conversational language, to reconcile this authoritative scientific position with a synthetic, 'pseudo-intimacy' with the reader.

In the Introduction to this chapter, we highlighted how CDA is interested in linking specific texts to their modes of production (meso-level) and wider social practices (macro-level) (Fairclough, 1992: 9). This 'linking' can include intertextual and interdiscursive relationships with other texts (see particularly Fairclough, 2013: 420–2). In labelling 'discourses' that occur in data, researchers are often faced with a practical challenge of how to name and link local discourses to these broader discourses. Some practical, step-wise approaches to this can be found in Wodak and Meyer (2001), although much of this will rest on the interpretation of the analyst.

9.3.4 Encouraging consumers to self-evaluate their hair loss

The strategy of 'pseudo-intimacy' with the reader links to the fourth discourse Harvey finds across the sites, *Encouraging consumers to self-evaluate their hair loss*, where questionnaires and self-diagnostic tools are employed to encourage website users to engage and see if they are 'eligible' to request Propecia. They are sometimes directed to use the 'Norwood-Hamilton Scale of male pattern baldness' (Figure 9.3). Harvey highlights that this is a classification system used in clinical contexts, by health professionals such as dermatologists, but which can be exploited here by these pharmaceutical websites to give a clinical legitimacy to the website user's hair loss concerns, linking to the use of scientific discourses above. This encourages self-diagnosis and the uptake of a pharmaceutical remedy.

9.4 Conclusions

This case study has focused on approaches you might take to looking at large scale societal 'discourses' or broad ideas from medical sociology, such as 'medicalization', to develop a systematic linguistics research project on a manageable scale. This can be achieved through identifying particular instances of the phenomenon in real-life practice (here, online advertising for hair loss remedies) and developing a principled means of selecting a workable dataset from the wealth of material that is often available.

Overall, Harvey's study presents an effective multimodal critical discourse analysis of the eight websites, making a convincing case for the four discourses his

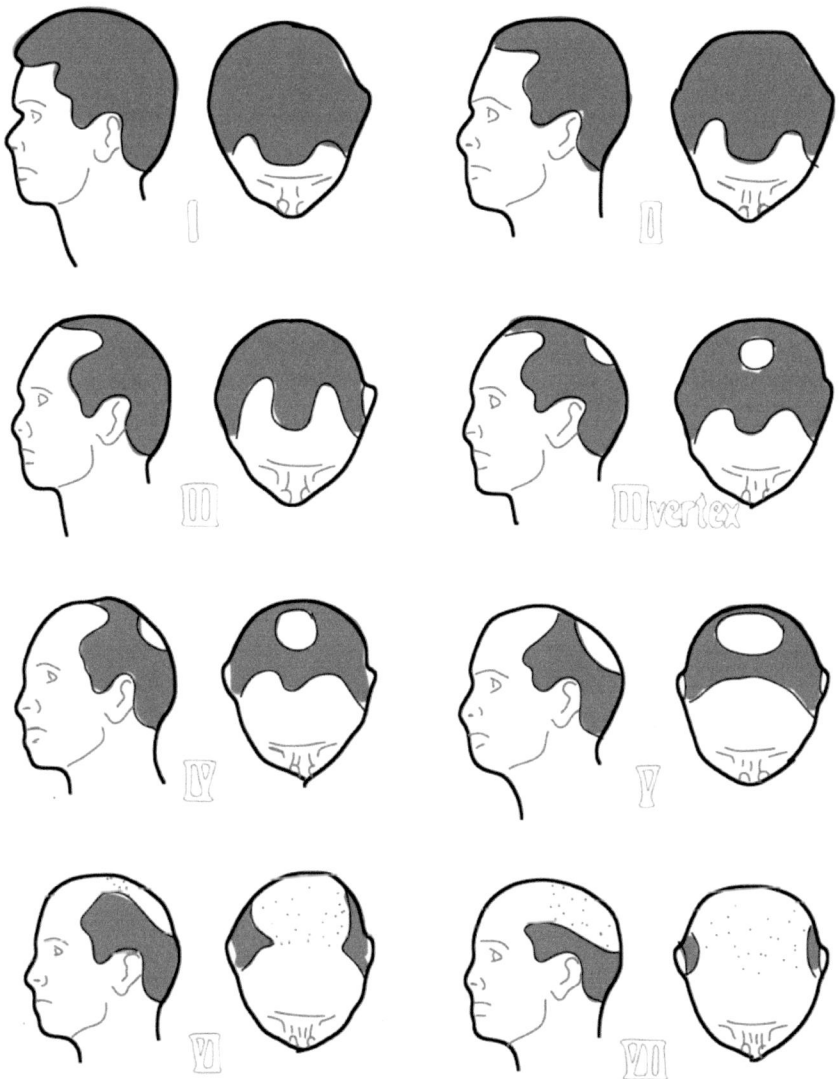

FIGURE 9.3   The Norwood–Hamilton Scale of male pattern baldness

study identified and the persuasive strategies used by pharmaceutical companies, particularly the appropriation of scientific discourses to promote a commercial product to the lay reader/viewer. For smaller scale studies, e.g. at Undergraduate or Masters level, even eight websites could constitute too much data so you may need to narrow your selection criteria even more (see Chapter 2). As indicated above, it can also be difficult to determine how many discourses you should identify across collections of texts and the limits to micro-textual strategies you should analyze as part of these. It is worth noting that researchers in this area generally take the view that, 'a complete discourse analysis of a large corpus of text or talk, as we often have in CDA research, is […] out of the question' (van Dijk, 2001: 99), and so the analysis need not necessarily be exhaustive but rather focus in on specific realizations of power and ideology that are relevant for the research questions you are trying to answer.

Multimodal elements of the text have become increasingly incorporated into critical discourse studies, addressing how the visual components of texts communicate with a viewer. The analysis here demonstrates how visual elements work to stigmatize baldness and represent an 'ideal', aspirational image of masculinity. As Harvey highlights though, the lexical/textual elements cannot be neglected, with MCDA requiring a careful analysis of the interplay between visual *and* textual elements. His MCDA analysis shows how textual and visual choices can be ideologically (and commercially) motivated and that close linguistic analysis such as this can do much to highlight the processes through which the phenomenon of 'medicalization' occurs through language, processes which have been largely overlooked in the medical sociology literature.

References

Bonaccorso, S., & Sturchio, J. (2002). Direct to consumer advertising is medicalising normal human experience. *British Medical Journal*, *324*, 910–911. https://doi.org/10.1136/bmj.324.7342.910

Brennan, R., Eagle, L., & Rice, D. (2009). Medicalization and marketing. *Journal of Macromarketing*, *30*(1), 8–22.

Conrad, P. (1992). Medicalization and social control. *Annual Review of Sociology*, *18*(1), 209–232.

Conrad, P. (2005). The shifting engines of medicalization. *Journal of Health and Social Behavior*, *45*, 158–176.

Conrad, P. (2007). *The medicalization of society: On the transformation of human conditions into treatable disorders*. Johns Hopkins University Press.

Ebrahim, S. (2002). The medicalisation of old age should be encouraged. *British Medical Journal*, *324*(7342), 861–863.

Fairclough, N. (1992). *Discourse and social change*. Polity Press.

Fairclough, N. (2001). *Language and power* (2nd ed.). Longman.

Fairclough, N. (2013). *Critical discourse analysis: The critical study of language* (2nd ed.). Routledge.

Fox, N., & Ward, K. (2008). Pharma in the bedroom … and the kitchen … The pharmaceuticalisation of daily life. *Sociology of Health and Illness*, *30*(6), 856–868.

Halliday, M. A. K., & Matthiessen, C. M. (2013). *Halliday's introduction to functional grammar* (4th ed.). Routledge.

Harvey, K. (2013). Medicalisation, pharmaceutical promotion and the Internet: A critical multimodal discourse analysis of hair loss websites. *Social Semiotics*, *23*(5), 691–714. https://doi.org/10.1080/10350330.2013.777596

Koteyko, N., & Nerlich, B. (2007). Multimodal discourse analysis of probiotic web advertising. *The International Journal of Language, Society and Culture*, *23*, 20–31.

Kress, G., & Van Leeuwen, T. (2020). *Reading images: The grammar of visual design*. Routledge.

Lovett, D. (2002). Using the web as a resource on hair loss. *Health Care on the Internet*, *6*(1–2), 99–109. https://doi.org/10.1300/J138v06n01_10

Mintzes, B. (2002). Direct to consumer advertising is medicalising normal human experience. *British Medical Journal*, *324*, 908–911. https://doi.org/10.1136/bmj.324 .7342.908

Moynihan, R., Heath, I., & Henry, D. (2002). Selling sickness: The pharmaceutical industry and disease mongering. *British Medical Journal*, *324*(7342), 886–890.

Nerlich, B., & Koteyko, N. (2008). Balancing food risks and food benefits: The coverage of probiotics in the UK national press. *Sociological Research Online*, *13*(3), 15–28. https://doi.org/10.5153/sro.1692

Thomas, F. (2021). Medicalisation. In K. Chamberlain & A. Lyons (Eds.), *Routledge international handbook of critical issues in health and illness* (1st ed., pp. 23–33). Routledge. https://doi.org/10.4324/9781003185215

van Dijk, T. (2001). Multidisciplinary cda: A plea for diversity. In T. van Dijk (Ed.), *Multidisciplinary CDA: A plea for diversity* (pp. 95–120). Sage. https://doi.org/10.4135 /9780857028020

Wodak, R., & Meyer, M. (Eds.). (2001). *Methods of critical discourse analysis*. Sage.

10

METAPHORS AND COVID-19 IN 2020

10.1 Introduction and rationale

What do wars, fires, hedgehogs, and glitter have in common? They were all used as metaphors for some aspect of the Covid-19 pandemic in the course of 2020, alongside many other concepts and phenomena. In fact, metaphor was so prominent in communication about the pandemic that it is now the topic of a very large number of studies involving different kinds of data, approaches and languages (e.g. volume 37.2 of the journal *Metaphor and Symbol*). In this chapter we discuss one of the first studies to be published in English on metaphors and Covid-19, by one of the three authors of this book: '"Not soldiers but fire-fighters" – Metaphors and Covid-19' (Semino, 2021). We show how this particular study addressed questions that arose unexpectedly and that involved ongoing and fast-developing events. This was achieved partly by drawing from relevant evidence provided in previous research and partly by analyzing data that was made available in a timely fashion in 2020, thanks to the generosity and collaborative efforts of a large number of researchers.

The origins of this study lie in the early months of the Covid-19 pandemic. When a new coronavirus was first identified as a possible cause of a serious form of pneumonia in China's Wuhan province in January 2020, many governments around the world underplayed the risks this would pose to their own populations. By March 2020, however, the virus was spreading so fast and with such serious consequences for people and health systems that country after country introduced the most stringent lockdown measures in living memory, requiring anybody other than people working in essential services not to leave their homes except in very limited circumstances (see also Chapter 4). It was notable, at that particular point, how metaphors to do with war were used by many political leaders to convey the gravity of the situation and justify the strict

DOI: 10.4324/9781003020417-13

measures that were being taken. In the USA, for example, President Donald Trump described himself as a 'wartime President' (The Guardian, 2020). In France, President Emmanuel Macron declared that 'Nous sommes en guerre, en guerre sanitaire' ('We are in a healthcare war') (Lemarié & Pietralunga, 2020). In the UK, on 17th March 2020, a statement by Prime Minister Boris Johnson included a War metaphor that Semino (2021: 50) uses to open her article:

> Yes this enemy can be deadly, but it is also beatable – and we know how to beat it and we know that if as a country we follow the scientific advice that is now being given we know that we will beat it.
> And however tough the months ahead we have the resolve and the resources to win the fight.

Semino points out how the use of these metaphors was widely noticed and criticized. Articles appeared in the media suggesting that War metaphors were inappropriate and should not be used (e.g. Tamkin, 2020). Researchers specializing in metaphor pointed out some well-evidenced shortcomings of War metaphors (e.g. Nerlich, 2020) and a group of scholars from Spain and the UK, including Semino, used Twitter in March 2020 to launch an appeal for the sharing of non-War metaphors for the pandemic, using the hashtag #ReframeCovid (Olza et al., 2021). At that time, members of the #ReframeCovid group and other specialists in the study of metaphor were regularly invited by the media to comment on the use of metaphors for Covid-19. What journalists wanted to know was not just what metaphors were being used and why, but also what metaphors *should* or *should not* be used, especially in view of criticisms of apparently dominant War metaphors. Semino's study was inspired by these questions, and brought together insights from previous research on metaphor and some new empirical findings in order to answer them.

10.1.1 *Key literature*

Semino defines metaphor as the phenomenon that involves talking and, potentially, thinking, about one thing in terms of another, where the two things are different but some similarities or correspondences can be perceived between them (see Chapter 8 for a method of metaphor identification). For example, the UK Prime Minister's statement mentioned above talks about the coronavirus as an enemy to be beaten. Viruses and enemies are different kinds of entities, but it is possible to perceive similarities between the new virus and an enemy: both are dangerous for individual lives and society, both require urgent action, and so on. This definition is placed in the context of three interconnected traditions in the study of metaphor, based, respectively, in the analysis of discourse (or naturally occurring language use), theories of cognition, and experimental psycholinguistic research.

The discourse perspective is represented by research that has pointed out the relatively high frequency of metaphor in language, ranging between 3 and 18 instances per 100 words (e.g. Cameron, 2003; Steen et al., 2010). This research is also concerned with the functions that metaphors perform in different types of communication, such as expressing subjective experiences (e.g. love as a flame), explaining difficult concepts (e.g. DNA as instructions written in our genes), and persuading others about particular evaluations or courses of action (e.g. immigrants as a flood).

The cognitive perspective has a long-standing tradition, but is particularly associated with Lakoff and Johnson's (1980) Conceptual Metaphor Theory. From this perspective, metaphorical expressions in discourse (e.g. 'I need a new direction in my life') are linguistic realizations of conceptual metaphors (e.g. LIFE IS A JOURNEY), which consist of mappings, or correspondences, from a 'source' conceptual domain (e.g. JOURNEY) to a 'target' conceptual domain (e.g. LIFE). Crucially, the choice of source domain affects the way in which the target domain is conceptualized, highlighting some aspects and backgrounding others – a process referred to as 'framing'. The LIFE IS A JOURNEY metaphor, for example, frames the achievement of goals in life as more important than contentedness with what one has. This is because, within that metaphor, purposes correspond to destinations, and, in a journey, reaching one's destination is preferable to standing still. The framing function of metaphor is also one of the reasons why it is of interest to researchers exploring its use and implications in discourse.

The experimental perspective aims to investigate whether and how metaphors have framing effects. For example, Hendricks et al. (2019) created two versions of a story about a person with cancer, one involving the metaphor of cancer as a battle, and the other involving the metaphor of cancer as a journey. Two groups of people read one or the other version of the story and then answered the same set of questions about the situation. Hendricks et al. found, among other things, that the people who read the Battle version of the text attributed greater feelings of guilt to the person if they did not get better than the people who read the Journey version. This was interpreted as evidence of a contrast in the framing effects of the two metaphors. In the Battle metaphor, not recovering corresponds to 'losing the battle', which can be due to not being strong or determined enough. No comparable guilt-inducing association applies to the Journey metaphor.

10.2 Methods and data

Semino's (2021) study was conducted in mid-to-late 2020 and first published online in November 2020 in the journal *Health Communication*, as part of a Special Issue on Public Health Communication in an Age of Covid-19. As it appeared in a scientific journal, it is primarily aimed at an academic readership, but it was not intended for specialists in metaphor and was written in such a way as to be understandable by as wide a readership as possible. Its stated aim is to discuss different metaphors for the pandemic, and explain 'why they are used and why they matter' (Semino, 2021: 51). It is structured around five specific questions:

1. Why is the pandemic talked about metaphorically?
2. Why are War metaphors in particular used for the pandemic?
3. Are the critics of War metaphors right to be concerned?
4. Should metaphors be avoided altogether?
5. Which metaphors should be used, and which avoided?

These questions were formulated in order to address concerns and debates that were highly topical in discussions of public communication in the early months of the pandemic in 2020. However, while Covid-19 was a new phenomenon, questions about where metaphors come from and how they should or should not be used were most definitely not new. Therefore, in the absence (at the time) of research findings on metaphors for Covid-19 specifically, the first four questions are answered by drawing from previous research on metaphor, including particularly War metaphors and metaphors in communication about illness. The use of War metaphors for illness, and for problems generally, was also not at all new. This illustrates how some research questions can be answered by referring to existing literature, while others require specific data to be analyzed and, often, collected.

The answer to the final question in Semino's study relies for the most part on evidence of metaphor use drawn from two Covid-specific datasets: the #ReframeCovid collection (https://sites.google.com/view/reframecovid/home) and the Coronavirus Corpus (www.english-corpora.org/corona/). Both already existed when Semino undertook the research.

The #ReframeCovid collection of metaphors was a new and rather unusual dataset, in that it was the result of a collaborative enterprise that relied on social media and an open-source online document where anyone could add examples of metaphors for the pandemic. Semino reports that, when she carried out her study, the collection included over 550 examples of (non-war) metaphors for different aspects of the pandemic, provided by approximately 100 people and involving 30 different languages and many different genres. All examples in the collection are classified by the person who enters them in terms of the source domain of the metaphor (Lakoff & Johnson, 1980), e.g. Sports for 'Covid-19 is a marathon, not a sprint'. Semino was therefore able to search the collection for metaphors drawing from different source domains in different languages, and specifically Fire metaphors, which, Semino argues, proved to be particularly useful at that point in the pandemic.

As a data source, such a collection has both strengths and weaknesses. On the one hand, it goes beyond what an individual researcher or team could realistically collect in the space of a few months. On the other hand, there was no explicit and systematic approach to data collection, which means that the metaphors included in the collection are rather heterogeneous and cannot be taken to be representative of metaphor use in any particular country, language, genre, or period of time. However, it was nonetheless appropriate and useful as a source of examples from different languages for Semino's study.

The Coronavirus Corpus was created as an addition to an influential and widely used collection of corpora of English available from www.english-corpora.org. It consists of news articles from 20 different countries (including UK, USA, Australia, India, Jamaica, etc.), harvested from the Web from 1st January 2020 onwards. At the time of writing (October 2022), it continues to grow by 3–4 million words per day. Semino's study is based on the corpus as of 30th September 2020, when it contained just over 600 million words. Unlike the #ReframeCovid collection, the Coronavirus Corpus is limited to one language and one genre. On the other hand, it is international and extremely large, and registration for a basic account is free.

The interface for the Coronavirus Corpus includes several of the tools typically associated with Corpus Linguistics, notably, a concordance tool and a collocation tool (see Chapter 2). To find a larger set of Fire metaphors (in English) than was available in the #ReframeCovid collections, Semino searched for the strings 'coronavirus' or 'covid-19' in a span five words to the left and five words to the right of the word 'fire'. She then examined each concordance line to determine whether it did indeed contain a fire-related metaphorical expression (according to the identification procedure by Pragglejaz Group 2007 mentioned in Chapter 8) or a simile that captured some aspect of the pandemic (e.g. 'the raging COVID-19 dumpster fire in the U.S.', as opposed to references to actual fires). This approach has the merit of efficiency, given the size of the corpus, but does not of course make it possible to identify Fire metaphors that do not involve the lexical item 'fire' (e.g. metaphorical uses of 'flames' or 'burn' in relation to the pandemic without 'fire' in close proximity).

Both data sources are used to provide empirical evidence of metaphor use during the pandemic, and to support a particular argument about metaphors of Covid-19 as a fire, namely that Fire metaphors 'are particularly appropriate and versatile in communication about different aspects of the pandemic' (Semino, 2021: 51). This claim is based on an analysis of the specific topics and functions of 61 instances of Fire metaphors: 7 from the #ReframeCovid collection in 6 languages (Dutch, English, German, Greek, Italian, and Spanish), and 54 instances from the Coronavirus Corpus, all in English.

10.3 Results and discussion

To answer the question 'Why is the pandemic talked about metaphorically?', Semino refers to the claim, made within Conceptual Metaphor Theory and beyond, that the experiences that typically function as target domains tend to be unfamiliar, abstract, complex, subjective, and/or sensitive. The Covid-19 pandemic had all of these characteristics: it was a new experience for most people alive at the time, it made daily life frightening and unrecognizable, it caused illness, distress, and death on an unprecedented scale, and had many different facets – medical, economic, social, and so on.

The more specific question 'Why are War metaphors in particular used for the pandemic?' is answered by pointing out a well known conventional metaphorical tendency, in English and other languages, to talk about problems as enemies. This tendency has been captured by Grady (1997) via the 'primary' metaphor DIFFICULTIES ARE OPPONENTS, which explains why experiences as varied as illness, debt, or grief can be 'struggled with,' 'fought,' and 'defeated.' From this perspective, it is not at all surprising that metaphors to do with physical fights and wars were used for the new coronavirus and the illness it caused.

Semino's third question 'Are the critics of War metaphors right to be concerned?' was less straightforward to answer. At that point, there was no evidence of people's reactions to War metaphors for the pandemic. Moreover, the appropriateness of using military language at all and the desirability of its possible effects are a matter of debate. However, Semino shows how the findings of previous research on the framing effects of War metaphors could go some way towards answering the question. In this case, as is often the case with metaphors generally, the answer was not clear-cut: 'Yes, the critics of War metaphors are right to be concerned, but War metaphors can also be useful'.

On the one hand, it has been found that War metaphors can increase people's perceptions of particular issues as serious and urgent, to the point that they are more willing to change their lifestyles to address them, as in the case of climate change (Flusberg et al., 2017; see also Chapter 4 on the issue of effectiveness of campaigns aiming to change people's views of behaviours). On the other hand, it has been found that, in the context of cancer prevention, War metaphors can increase fatalism and decrease people's willingness to refrain from behaviours that are associated with higher cancer risks, such as smoking (Hauser & Schwarz, 2015, 2020). Both kinds of findings were potentially relevant to the context of the pandemic. On the one hand, they suggest that, setting aside any moral objections to the use of military language, War metaphors may have indeed been useful at the start of the pandemic to persuade people that the new coronavirus posed a very serious threat and required major changes in individual and collective behaviour. On the other hand, War metaphors may have been less appropriate to justify the unprecedented restraint that many people had to exercise by staying at home. In addition, a fatalistic attitude towards the possibility of controlling the pandemic could have undermined compliance in the long run, especially when the metaphorical war became protracted over months and years. Indeed, even though War metaphors continued to be used throughout the pandemic, there is some evidence that, on Twitter, their frequency declined after the first few months (Wicke & Bolognesi, 2021).

Semino's last two questions – 'Should metaphors be avoided altogether?' and 'Which metaphors should be used, and which avoided?' – are not the kind of questions that linguistic researchers tend to be directly concerned with. Metaphor scholars, for example, typically theorize, describe, and/or critique metaphor use, but do not aim to prescribe behaviour. However, questions such as these have been regularly asked by many people, from philosophers to journalists, especially when faced with uses of metaphors they found objectionable. And these precise questions were being asked in the early months of the pandemic, including, for example, by journalists interviewing members of the #ReframeCovid group.

With regard to whether metaphors should be avoided altogether, on the grounds that they can be harmful, Semino makes reference to previous studies, particularly on metaphors for cancer, to argue that this is neither possible nor desirable (see also Chapter 8). It is not possible because, as suggested by Conceptual Metaphor Theory, thinking and talking through metaphors are central human tendencies and abilities, to the extent that we are often not conscious that we are reasoning or communicating through metaphors. But avoiding metaphors altogether is also not desirable because metaphors can do good as well as harm, and dispensing with them would considerably limit the scope, depth, and creativity of our communication and reasoning. What matters, Semino argues, is not whether metaphors should be used, but *how* they are used. This requires a consideration of contexts, audiences, and purposes. In the presence of a new and serious danger, for example, even War metaphors may be argued to have their uses, in spite of their considerable downsides.

More generally, however, Semino points out that a variety of different metaphors are needed when faced with complex and long-standing problems such as a global pandemic, as each metaphor can only capture *part* of a particular phenomenon, and from a particular perspective. The #ReframeCovid collection is used to demonstrate this point.

Journey metaphors, for example, can be used to present the pandemic as a long and difficult process, requiring patience and resilience, such as when the President of Bavaria said, in April 2020: 'Daher sind wir noch nicht über den Berg' ('That's why we're not over the mountain-[top] yet'). Metaphors to do with natural disasters are particularly effective when trying to convey the effects of the pandemic on health services, for example in terms of tsunamis and avalanches. More creative metaphors may be needed, however, for some very specific audiences and purposes. Describing the virus as 'glitter' that 'gets everywhere' makes a serious point about the virus's invisibility in a light-hearted manner, and may be particularly appropriate for children. Capturing the particular type of sacrifice and endurance involved in staying at home also requires new, creative metaphors. A Norwegian example in the #ReframeCovid collection describes the specific 'heroism' demanded of people during lockdowns as 'gjøre som pinnsvinet' ('acting like a hedgehog'), i.e. 'rulle seg sammen og vente, håper på bedre tider' ('roll up in a ball and wait, hope for better times'). This contrasts with the intense activity that is associated with more prototypical types of heroism, for example in war (see also Pérez-Sobrino et al., 2022).

Having said all this, Semino argues that it is possible to use multiple sources of evidence to make a case that some metaphors may be more useful and appropriate for a specific phenomenon than others, and exemplifies this with reference to Fire metaphors and the pandemic.

Previous research suggests that, to be effective, metaphors need to involve, among other things: (1) widely accessible, well delineated, and image-rich source domains; and (2) precise and clearly applicable mappings, or correspondences, from source to target domain (Grady, 2017, Thibodeau et al., 2017). As a source domain, Fire fulfils criterion 1. Fires are vivid and familiar, even if mostly experienced second hand. They can be of different kinds (e.g. forest fires, house fires). They involve many different aspects (e.g. objects, arsonists, victims, fire-fighters). And they evolve, i.e. they start, peak, and end. As such, they are conventionally used for negative phenomena that we perceive as 'spreading' (Charteris-Black, 2017, Hart, 2017), and a contagious illness is one of these phenomena. Indeed, there are clear correspondences between fires and pandemics (criterion 2), for example, between the virus and flames, and healthcare professionals or scientists as fire-fighters.

The 61 examples of Fire metaphors drawn from the #ReframeCovid collection and the Coronavirus Corpus are used by Semino to provide evidence of the different functions that Fire metaphors were used to perform in the first months of the pandemic. These functions include:

Convey danger and urgency – e.g. the pandemic as, in Spanish, 'un gran fuego' ('a large fire') or a 'forest fire that may not slow down'.

Distinguish between different phases of the pandemic – e.g. the coronavirus as a 'fire raging' when prevalence is high vs. trying to 'find any burning embers of the virus' when prevalence is low.

Explain how contagion happens and how to reduce it – e.g. this extract from a piece in the medical information website Medscape:

Think of COVID-19 as a fire burning in a forest. All of us are trees. The R0 is the wind speed. The higher it is, the faster the fire tears through the forest.

But just like a forest fire, COVID-19 needs fuel to keep going. We're the fuel.

If the R0 is low enough, the fire stays in one place and burns itself out; we don't all get infected. A few fire lines—quarantines and social distancing measures—keep the fire from hitting all the trees.

(Wilson, 2020)

Connect the pandemic with health inequalities and other problems – e.g. the coronavirus 'add[ing] fuel to the fire' or 'throw[ing] gasoline on the fire' in the context of pre-existing tensions in US prisons or of long-term mental health problems.

Outline post-pandemic futures – e.g. the idea of 'reclaiming the soil' after a fire in this Italian example from the #ReframeCovid collection:

Non solo ci sono continuamente focolai da spegnere e, quando la sorte si accanisce, giganteschi fronti di fuoco da arginare, ma è dovere di tutti collaborare quotidianamente alla bonifica del terreno affinché scintille, inneschi, distrazioni più o meno colpevoli non provochino adesso o in futuro disastri irreparabili.

Not only are there constant outbreaks to extinguish and, when our luck gets worse, gigantic fronts of fire to control, but it is everyone's duty to collaborate daily in the reclamation of the soil, so that sparks, triggers, and more or less guilty distractions do not cause irreparable disasters now or in the future. (Costa, 2020)

This variety of functions is used by Semino as evidence of the versatility of Fire metaphors to capture different aspects of the pandemic. The precision of the correspondences in each case is used as evidence of appropriateness, e.g. between low infections and embers, infected people and burning trees, social distancing, and fire lines, and so on.

Semino also points out, however, the inevitable limitations of Fire metaphors (e.g. not easily accounting for asymptomatic transmission) and emphasizes that, while some metaphors are more useful than others, a variety of metaphors will always be needed for something as complex and persistent as a global pandemic.

10.4 Conclusions

The study we have discussed in this chapter is part of a well-established tradition of research on metaphor in communication about illness (Demjén & Semino, 2017, Tay, 2017). In this respect, there is huge potential for further work, and many models of good practice in the identification and analysis of metaphors in different kinds of data and through different kinds of methods (e.g. Maslen, 2017, Nacey et al., 2019).

In addition, Semino's paper is also an example of how linguistic studies can respond to public health challenges as they unfold. As such, it shows how, in some cases, it is possible to answer questions about a new phenomenon by drawing from the findings of relevant existing research that may not be on the same topic, but has some things in common. Furthermore, it is possible and sometimes necessary to use empirical evidence from general data sources, when they are available. The timely creation of both the #ReframeCovid collection and the Coronavirus Corpus were indeed essential to Semino's study. In particular, the crowdsourcing and sharing of linguistic examples that resulted in the #ReframeCovid collection will hopefully be a growing part of how researchers operate in future, privileging collaboration over competition.

Researching an aspect of a fast-developing crisis also involves risks, however, for example if hoped-for data does not materialize or if a new development challenges an analysis while it is in progress (see also Chapter 11). This needs to be taken into account when planning projects with short timescales and unmoveable deadlines. However, with appropriate planning, there can be considerable rewards in tackling extremely current topics, and the potential to make a positive contribution to society.

References

Cameron, L. (2003). *Metaphor in educational discourse*. Continuum.

Charteris-Black, J. (2017). *Fire metaphors: Discourses of awe and authority*. Bloomsbury.

Costa, P. (2020). Emergenza coronavirus: Non soldati, ma pompieri. *Settimana News*. Retrieved October 9, 2022, from http://www.settimananews.it/societa/emergenza -coronavirus-non-soldati-ma-pompieri/

Demjén, Z., & Semino, E. (2017). Using metaphor in healthcare: Physical health. In E. Semino & Z. Demjén (Eds.), *The Routledge handbook of metaphor and language* (pp. 385–399). Routledge.

Flusberg, S. J., Matlock, T., & Thibodeau, P. H. (2017). Metaphors for the war (or race) against climate change. *Environmental Communication*, *11*(6), 769–783.

Grady, J. (1997). Theories are buildings revisited. *Cognitive Linguistics*, *8*(4), 267–290.

Grady, J. (2017). Using metaphor to influence public perceptions and policy: How metaphors can save the world. In E. Semino & Z. Demjén (Eds.), *The Routledge handbook of metaphor and language* (pp. 343–354). Routledge.

The Guardian. (2020). 'Invisible enemy': Trump says he is 'wartime president' in coronavirus battle. Retrieved October 9, 2022, from https://www.theguardian.com/ world/video/2020/mar/23/invisible-enemy-trump-says-he-is-wartime-president-in -coronavirus-battle-video

Hart, C. (2017). "Riots engulfed the city": An experimental study investigating the legitimating effects of fire metaphors in discourses of disorder. *Discourse and Society*, *29*(3), 279–298.

Hauser, D. J., & Schwarz, N. (2015). The war on prevention: Bellicose cancer metaphors hurt (some) prevention intentions. *Personality and Social Psychology Bulletin*, *41*(1), 66–77.

Hauser, D. J., & Schwarz, N. (2020). The war on prevention II: Battle metaphors undermine cancer treatment and prevention and do not increase vigilance. *Health Communication*, *35*(13), 1698–1704.

Hendricks, R. K., Demjén, Z., Semino, E., & Boroditsky, L. (2019). Emotional implications of metaphor: Consequences of metaphor framing for mindset about cancer. *Metaphor and Symbol*, *33*(4), 267–279.

Lakoff, G., & Johnson, M. (1980). *Metaphors we live by*. University of Chicago Press.

Lemarié, A., & Pietralunga, C. (2020). 'Nous sommes en guerre': Face au coronavirus, Emmanuel Macron sonne la 'mobilisation générale'. *Le Monde*. Retrieved October 9, 2022, from https://www.lemonde.fr/politique/article/2020/03/17/nous-sommes-en -guerre-face-au-coronavirus-emmanuel-macron-sonne-la-mobilisation-generale _6033338_823448.html

Maslen, R. (2017). Finding systematic metaphors. In E. Semino & Z. Demjén (Eds.), *The Routledge handbook of metaphor and language* (pp. 88–101). Routledge.

Nacey, S., Dorst, A. G., Krennmayr, T., & Reijnierse, W. G. (2019). *Metaphor identification in multiple languages: MIPVU around the world*. John Benjamins.

Nerlich, B. (2020, September 18). Metaphors and realities: Coronavirus and climate change. Retrieved October 9, 2022, from https://blogs.nottingham.ac.uk/ makingsciencepublic/2020/09/18/metaphors-and-realities-coronavirus-and-climate -change/

Olza, I., Koller, V., Ibarretxe-Antuñano, I., Pérez-Sobrino, P., & Semino, E. (2021). The #ReframeCovid initiative: From Twitter to society via metaphor. *Metaphor and the Social World, 11*(1), 98–120.

Pérez-Sobrino, P., Semino, E., Ibarretxe-Antuñano, I., Koller, V., & Olza, I. (2022). Acting like a hedgehog in times of pandemic: Metaphorical creativity in the #ReframeCovid collection. *Metaphor and Symbol, 37*(2), 127–139.

Semino, E. 'Not soldiers but fire-fighters': Metaphors and Covid-19. *Health Communication, 36*(1), 50–58.

Steen, G. J., Dorst, A. G., Herrmann, B. J., Kaal, A. A., Krennmayr, T., & Pasma, T. (2010). *A method for linguistic metaphor identification: From MIP to MIPVU.* John Benjamins.

Tamkin, E. (2020). Using military language to discuss coronavirus is dangerous and irresponsible – The US must stop. *New Statesman.* Retrieved from October 9, 2022, https://www.newstatesman.com/world/north-america/2020/04/using-military-language-discuss-coronavirus-dangerous-and-irresponsible

Tay, D. (2017). Using metaphor in healthcare: Mental health. In E. Semino & Z. Demjén (Eds.), *The Routledge handbook of metaphor and language* (pp. 371–384). Routledge.

Thibodeau, P. H., Hendricks, R. K., & Boroditsky, L. (2017). How linguistic metaphor scaffolds reasoning. *Trends in Cognitive Sciences, 21*(11), 852–863.

Wicke, P., & Bolognesi, M. (2021). Covid-19 discourse on Twitter: How the topics, sentiments, subjectivity, and figurative frames changed over time. *Frontiers in Communication, 6*, 1–20.

Wilson, F. P. (2020, March 31). COVID-19 death predictions: What do we need to know? *Medscape.* Retrieved October 9, 2022, from https://www.medscape.com/viewarticle/927791

11
VACCINATION NARRATIVES IN RESPONSE TO HESITANCY ONLINE

11.1 Introduction

Vaccination programmes are a major success story, estimated to have prevented around 2–3 million deaths a year worldwide even before the Covid-19 pandemic (WHO, 2019). Yet, around the world there is also resistance to vaccinations. In this chapter, we showcase the study 'Pro-vaccination personal narratives in response to online hesitancy about the HPV vaccine: The challenge of tellability' by Semino et al. (in press). This study was conducted as part of a large, funded research project on vaccination discourses that two of the authors (ZD and ES) are involved in at the time of writing: 'Questioning Vaccination Discourse: a corpus-based approach'[1] (Quo Vadis, for short). Quo Vadis collected online language data related to vaccinations (among other sources) and faced a common problem in language research: having a lot of data and needing to identify specific foci. In this chapter, we discuss the process of how the team homed in on one such focus – the kinds of narratives that people post online in response to someone expressing reservations about vaccinating their child against the Human Papillomavirus (HPV). We show how even a 'big data' study can be narrowed down to a scale that is possible to analyze via manual intensive qualitative methods.

11.1.1 Why study vaccination discourses?

Vaccine hesitancy – defined by the World Health Organization (WHO) as 'a delay in acceptance or refusal of vaccines despite availability of vaccination services' – affects vaccination programmes in 90% of countries in the world and was listed as one of the WHO's ten global health threats in 2019 (WHO, 2019). In England, Romania, Germany, France, the United States, Philippines, and Samoa,

DOI: 10.4324/9781003020417-14

for example, the uptake of routine childhood vaccinations is in decline, and has led to outbreaks in communicable diseases, such as measles, that had previously been considered eradicated (Hotez et al., 2020). Vaccine hesitancy is not new, of course; it has a history as long as vaccinations themselves. However, the rapid, self-organizing manner in which anti-vaccination and vaccine hesitant views can be shared and amplified in public and private spaces online across geographical boundaries means that they can reach and influence more people, quicker than ever.

There has been a lot of research on the complex and multifaceted reasons for vaccine hesitancy. Most widely known is the belief in a causal link between the measles/mumps/rubella vaccine (MMR) and autism. This view persists among some people worldwide despite the original study suggesting this link being retracted and contradicted by several subsequent large-scale studies (e.g. Taylor et al., 2014). Some people also decide to delay or reject vaccinations due to beliefs that vaccines are toxic, that they primarily benefit pharmaceutical companies, that it is safer to acquire immunity via the illness itself, and so on. These beliefs are often part of a range of broader religious and/or political world views that, in different ways and for different reasons, may favour 'natural' lifestyles, are suspicious of multinational companies and/or question mainstream science and expertise (Fournet et al., 2018).

The expression of vaccine hesitancy, however, i.e. how it is raised and responded to in spontaneous interactions and discussions among peers, is far less well understood. In this context Quo Vadis aimed to be the first large-scale diachronic linguistic study of vaccination discourse in English, using the mixed-methods associated with corpus-based discourse analysis, which you have seen in Chapters 2, 7, and 8. The project focused on childhood vaccinations and both UK-specific and international data in English to provide in-depth and nuanced accounts of historical and current pro- and anti-vaccination views, arguments, and communication strategies. This is captured in the overarching research question of the project: *How are views about vaccinations expressed in public discourse in English, and what does this reveal about the causes of vaccine hesitancy and the ways in which they can be addressed in public health initiatives?*

The team planned to answer this question by examining views about vaccinations (e.g. beliefs, emotions, and attitudes) expressed and justified in:

- English-language contributions to three social media platforms: Twitter, Reddit, and Mumsnet, since the inception of each platform;
- UK national newspapers since 1990;
- UK parliamentary debates since 1830.

Each of these data types would be a corpus of its own, with possible subcorpora (e.g. according to time-period or online platform) within them, and would be examined using a range of corpus linguistic techniques.

Once the project got going, the overarching research question would need to be broken down into narrower, more focused questions, each contributing towards the objectives of the project. This is very common for research projects, especially large ones, where research aims and questions get formulated in relatively broad terms initially, requiring more specific operationalizations when the projects are carried out. Although dissertations and theses are on a relatively smaller scale, a similar process applies as students move from the proposal stage to actually carrying out their studies. The larger the project, the more specific foci and research questions you will need (see Chapter 2).

11.2 Identifying a focus for qualitative investigation within a large-scale dataset

In the next sections, we illustrate how the Quo Vadis team arrived at the decision to focus on narratives in response to hesitancy regarding the HPV vaccination on the parenting website Mumsnet.

11.2.1 Where to start?

Since the core focus of Quo Vadis was on childhood vaccinations, the team prioritized data collection from Mumsnet, a UK-based parenting website, as soon as the project began. Social media plays an important role in what people read about vaccinations (Wilson & Wiysonge, 2020) and parenting websites and community forums in particular are accessed as sources of information and spaces for interaction about childhood vaccinations, as well as vaccinations more generally. In fact, 29% of participants who used the internet to find out about vaccinations in Campbell et al.'s (2017) survey of parents in England specifically cited Mumsnet as a website they accessed for that purpose, with a smaller proportion citing Facebook or Twitter (13% for each platform).

Mumsnet hosts a popular community forum, Mumsnet Talk, which includes numerous threads discussing vaccinations. Quo Vadis collected all threads on Mumsnet Talk, where the original post (OP), i.e. the first post that starts a thread, used some version of the lemma vaccin* or jab* between 2000 and mid-2021. This resulted in a corpus of 12,288 threads amounting to over 31-million words. Although this corpus only made up a small part of the whole Quo Vadis dataset, it was already large-scale, and the team needed to identify a specific focus that would contribute to answering the overarching research question of the project.

The Quo Vadis team included a co-investigator from a UK public health agency who suggested that the HPV vaccine was of most interest to healthcare practitioners and policy makers. This was confirmed in conversations with a wider network of clinical academics – people who work as academics at universities, but are also practising clinicians. HPV is a virus typically transmitted through sexual contact, with certain strains causing serious conditions, including cervical cancer. Vaccination against HPV has been found to reduce the rates of cervical cancer by up to 87% (Falcaro et al., 2021), but the uptake of this vaccination is globally very low (Spayne & Hesketh, 2021). This suggests that HPV vaccination is particularly affected by vaccine hesitancy. Given the interest of healthcare professionals, and the fact that the HPV vaccine is a childhood vaccine and therefore core to the Quo Vadis project aims, the team decided to prioritize a focus on discussions of HPV vaccine hesitancy on Mumsnet.

There are, of course, many aspects of HPV vaccine hesitancy on Mumsnet that could be explored so the Quo Vadis team next took inspiration from a specific debate in the literature about the usefulness of information versus narratives in countering anti-vaccination or vaccine hesitant views. In the next section we briefly outline this debate.

11.2.2 Zooming in on narratives

People often assume that vaccine hesitancy (and indeed the outright rejection of vaccinations) is a result of not having enough or the right kind of information. Information in this context usually means scientific facts and statistics. However, there is mounting evidence that people who are hesitant about, or against vaccinations are not short on information, and that additional facts or statistics are not particularly effective at changing their minds. Cawkell et al. (2016), for example, suggest that evidence from clinical findings about vaccines, including their safety, is not nearly as persuasive as the highly emotional narratives of vaccine harm. On the other hand, Nan et al. (2015) found that, when statistics were combined with narratives of HPV infection and abnormal cervical smear tests, especially those told in first-person, people saw infection as riskier and were therefore more open to being vaccinated to prevent it. Narratives or stories are often contrasted with 'information' as an alternative persuasive strategy in these studies, or with different types of narratives (e.g. first vs. third person; vaccine harm vs. vaccine safety).

From a theoretical perspective, narratives are thought to engage people differently, both in terms of cultural significance and cognitive processing. They are thought to create the conditions for immersion in a story world, identification with characters and increased emotional involvement, which may be able to bypass people's resistance to persuasion. As indicated above, however, there are many different types of stories and many ways to tell them, so a lot of experimental research and debate in this area is focused on understanding what kinds of stories are most likely to persuade people to take up vaccinations when they are offered (Ratcliff & Sun, 2020).

However, this experimental work cannot account for what stories are actually told spontaneously 'in the real world' and how. And some types of stories might be inherently less engaging or harder to tell in real world contexts. For example, when vaccinations prevent infections and illnesses without dramatic side-effects, there is very little from which to create a story. As most definitions of 'narrative' demonstrate, a story centres around some kind of 'complicating action' (Labov, 1972), something happening (see also section 8.3.3 in Chapter 8). But the point of successful and safe vaccination is precisely that nothing happens; there are no or only minor side-effects and no illness. This poses a challenge to good story-telling, because stories need to be 'tellable'. 'Tellability' is what makes the events in a narrative worth telling in a particular context (Labov, 1972). The problem is that, if successful vaccination does not lend itself to telling an engaging story, then there is unlikely to be a persuasive advantage to the narrative.

In the next section we describe how the Quo Vadis team identified sections of the 31-million word Mumsnet corpus relevant to exploring HPV vaccine hesitancy and the role of narratives.

11.3 Methods and narrowing down the data

If you have a large amount of potential data, but have narrowed down your scope, then the next crucial step is to somehow operationalize your scope, i.e. develop a systematic, principled, and replicable way of finding, for example, Mumsnet posts that will be most relevant to HPV vaccination, hesitancy, and narratives. This is often an iterative process, meaning that you narrow down in successive steps until you have a dataset that is appropriate to your aims and practical constraints (e.g. time and word-count). In the case of Quo Vadis, the 31-million word Mumsnet corpus was already focused on vaccinations: all threads included in the corpus started with an original post that mentioned vaccination in some way. The team just needed to identify threads discussing the HPV vaccine and expressing hesitancy.

Using corpus tools, the team searched the corpus for original posts that included the words 'hpv' or 'human papillomavirus'. The assumption was that if the OP of a thread is about HPV, then the replies and discussions following it are also likely to be (largely) about HPV. The researchers found 130 OPs that mentioned one or both of the search terms. They then screened the OPs to identify those that expressed hesitancy or indecision around the vaccination. This resulted in 25 relevant OPs (and therefore 25 threads) involving indecision or hesitancy about whether or not to accept an HPV vaccination (for a child), which brand of vaccine to accept, and whether or not to delay the vaccination.

Twenty-five threads on HPV vaccine hesitancy still represented a lot of data for an analysis of narratives or stories, which is necessarily qualitative, as threads can consist of hundreds of posts. The team noticed that, in 5 of these 25 threads, the user who wrote the original post returned to the thread after some of the discussion had taken place and announced the conclusion they had come to: to vaccinate (three cases) or not (two cases). In one of these cases, the original poster explicitly said that a particular narrative response, an excerpt of which is in Example 11.3, had led to her decision to allow their child to be vaccinated. This illustrates the element of serendipity that is always part of research projects: there are times when you can (and have to) operationalize concepts a priori. In other words, you decide before you begin your data collection how you will capture the effect or phenomenon you are interested in. But there are also times when an initial trawl through the data provides you with an alternative.

There are, of course, caveats here: the method outlined above does not identify all threads on HPV vaccine hesitancy that resulted in a decision on the part of the original poster, nor ones where this decision was based on a narrative reply. It only finds threads where such a decision was made public. It is also not possible, with this method, to ascertain whether those original posters did in fact allow their children to be, or prevent them from being, vaccinated. These caveats, however, do not mean that the data are not valuable or not representative. It is simply the case that the nature of the data needs to be borne in mind whenever interpretations are made and conclusions discussed. This is good practice for any research project. Most research investigating the persuasive power of narratives, including those introduced earlier for example, rely on controlled experiments and/or surveys. They have the advantage of large numbers of participants, but they do not uncover what, if any, narratives are actually told in response to expressions of vaccine hesitancy or indecision, nor how people respond to each other's stories 'in the wild'. The study discussed here is far less controlled, and includes only one case study thread (though this still involves 207 replies). But it has the advantage that it can explore discourse as it naturally unfolds in one particular context.

The method described above also illustrates how seamlessly quantitative and qualitative methods can be brought together. In fact, while Quo Vadis is primarily a corpus linguistic project dealing with 'big data', there are ways to narrow down and focus on certain aspects or parts of the data in qualitative, in-depth ways. As outlined above and in what follows, once the team had used corpus tools to identify the 130 OPs that referred to HPV, the rest of the analysis for this particular study proceeded qualitatively.

The thread involving HPV indecision, which also announced a decision based on a narrative reply, was extracted from the main corpus and the Quo Vadis team coded all replies to the OP to see whether they included information and/or narratives. In this chapter we focus on the replies that included narratives. Full narratives for this purpose were defined as 'the telling of at least two interconnected actions or events, not necessarily in chronological order' (Semino et al., in press). For example:

EXAMPLE 11.1

DD1 [*dear daughter 1*] had hers, after a bit of plea bargaining, she hates needles. We agreed she'd have her HPV and I'd let her off her flu one. She's on the list for ridiculously mild asthma and reacts really badly to them (gets a really painful arm for a week, HPV didn't bother her at all).

This example includes a discussion between parent/mother and daughter, the agreement that the daughter would have the HPV vaccine and not the flu vaccine, the uptake of the HPV vaccine, and, to include negated events, the absence of post-HPV-vaccination side-effects. These are presented as interconnected events, making this a narrative. The team also coded as 'narrative report' any posts that reported a single action or event, sometimes accompanied by some form of explanation or evaluation such as:

EXAMPLE 11.2

'My daughter has had the vaccine. I'd rather her be safe(r) than sorry'.

In the next section we summarize the findings in relation to narratives encouraging vaccination that are potentially most engaging and persuasive, but also difficult and risky to tell.

11.4 Results

Narrative responses to the OP encouraging them to allow their child to be vaccinated immediately (rather than refusing or delaying it to a later point) tended to centre either on experiences with the vaccine itself (Example 11.1 and Example 11.2 above) or with the health issues that the vaccine is intended to prevent as in Example 11.3:

EXAMPLE 11.3

I didn't have sex until I was 22, never smoked, was a veggie health freak, 2 boyfriends, regular smears. And hey presto by 30 I had what they call 'carcinoma in situ' and had 2 big chunks of my cervix cut out. Luckily I was able to have 2 kids afterwards but ended up with a hysterectomy at 35 as the remaining cells were starting to change.

Returning now to the idea of some stories being more engaging and 'tellable' than others, it is important to point out that tellability is partly a property of events themselves. Some events (e.g. illness) are inherently more tellable than others (e.g. uneventful vaccinations). However, the way in which events are told also impacts how tellable a narrative may appear. Overall, tellability is best seen as a vertical cline, with context-dependent thresholds between events that are too mundane to be turned into an engaging narrative at the lower end, events that make good narrative material or can be told engagingly (and therefore are more likely to be persuasive) in the middle, and events that are too sensitive, personal, or taboo to be tellable in most contexts (Norrick, 2005) at the upper end of the cline.

   The narratives revolving around vaccine uptake had to negotiate the lower threshold of the cline of tellability. Nothing exciting happens so there is not much out of which to create a story. These stories were either minimally narrative such as the narrative report in Example 11.2, or, on the more fully formed narrative side, were embellished with complicating events and emotions leading up to the actual vaccination, as in Example 11.1. These additional elements contribute to tellability by presenting obstacles to the uptake of vaccination that need to be overcome: a conflict between parent and daughter, and the unrealized possibility of a bad reaction to the vaccine that happened with previous vaccines but not with the HPV one.

Pro-vaccination stories that revolved around illness (such as Example 11.3) did not suffer from inherently less tellable material. Instead, they sometimes pushed at the upper threshold of the cline, with the events described being very personal and sometimes taboo, as HPV affects the reproductive organs. Telling these types of stories carries risks of personal exposure on the part of those who volunteer them (although these are somewhat mitigated by the anonymity of the online environment). In Example 11.3, a small excerpt from a much longer post, which ultimately led to the OP deciding to allow their child to be vaccinated, references to serious illness and its treatment involving the reproductive organs are risky, and approaching the upper boundary of tellability, especially because of associations between contracting HPV and irresponsible sexual activity. In fact, the writer of this post begins by acknowledging this difficult balancing act in saying that they 'thought long and hard about what to write on this thread' as it is 'quite difficult'.

The idea that it might actually be difficulty and personally risky – due to issues of tellability – to tell engaging pro-vaccination narratives is the type of insight into the 'how' of storytelling in response to vaccine indecision that cannot be arrived at in quantitative or experimental studies.

This insight implies that the use of such narratives in encouraging vaccine hesitant people to vaccinate cannot be recommended without reservations.

11.5 Conclusions

In this chapter we demonstrated how even a 'big data' study can be narrowed down to a scale that is possible to analyze via manual intensive qualitative coding and what the advantages of doing so might be. Most student and early-career researchers will face the problem of too big a topic or too much data. Inspiration for narrowing things down can come from a range of sources, but it is important to do it systematically, in a principled manner, while also bearing in mind practical constraints. This chapter has demonstrated a few ways of doing this.

Another point we wanted to emphasize is that while having a lot of data can be a good thing, it is not an advantage for all topics of interest. And even within big data there is room for qualitative work. Most research done on the persuasiveness of different types of narratives is experimental and often quantitative in nature. But it leaves a gap. It does not help to uncover what narratives are actually volunteered and how they are engaged with 'in the wild'. It could not possibly point towards a challenge of tellability, i.e. the difficulties of telling engaging stories of successful and safe vaccines. Better understanding these challenges can inform initiatives aimed at counteracting the claims and tactics that are driving down vaccination rates.

Note

1 Questioning Vaccination Discourses: a corpus-based study is based at Lancaster University and funded by the Economic and Social Research Council in the United Kingdom (ES/V000926/1).

References

Campbell, H., Edwards, A., Letley, L., Bedford, H., Ramsay, M., & Yarwood, J. (2017). Changing attitudes to childhood immunisation in English parents. *Vaccine*, *35*(22), 2979–2985.

Cawkwell, P. B., & Oshinsky, D. (2016). Storytelling in the context of vaccine refusal: A strategy to improve communication and immunisation. *Medical Humanities*, *42*(1), 31–35.

Falcaro, M., Castañon, A., Ndlela, B., Checchi, M., Soldan, K., Lopez-Bernal, J., . . . Sasieni, P. (2021). The effects of the national HPV vaccination programme in England, UK, on cervical cancer and grade 3 cervical intraepithelial neoplasia incidence: A register-based observational study. *The Lancet*, *398*(10316), 2084–2092.

Fournet, N., Mollema, L., Ruijs, W. L., Harmsen, I. A., Keck, F., Durand, J. Y., Cunha, M. P., Wamsiedel, M., Reis, R., French, J., Smit, E. G., Kitching, A. & van Steenbergen, J. E. (2018). Under-vaccinated groups in Europe and their beliefs, attitudes and reasons for non-vaccination; two systematic reviews. *BMC Public Health*, *18*(1), 196.

Hotez, P. J., Nuzhath, T., & Colwell, B. (2020). Combating vaccine hesitancy and other 21st century social determinants in the global fight against measles. *Current Opinion in Virology*, *41*, 1–7.

Labov, W. (1972). The transformation of experience in narrative syntax. In W. Labov (Ed.), *Language in the inner city: Studies in the Black English vernacular* (pp. 354–396). University of Pennsylvania Press.

Nan, X., Dahlstrom, M. F., Richards, A., & Rangarajan, S. (2015). Influence of evidence type and narrative type on HPV risk perception and intention to obtain the HPV vaccine. *Health Communication*, *30*(3), 301–308.

Norrick, N. (2005) The dark side of tellability. *Narrative Inquiry*, 15(2), 323–345

Ratcliff, C. L., & Sun, Y. (2020). Overcoming resistance through narratives: Findings from a meta-analytic review. *Human Communication Research*, *46*(4), 412–443.

Spayne, J., & Hesketh, T. (2021). Estimate of global human papillomavirus vaccination coverage: Analysis of country-level indicators. *BMJ Open*, *11*(9), e052016.

Taylor, L. E., Swerdfeger, A. L., & Eslick, G. D. (2014). Vaccines are not associated with autism: An evidence-based meta-analysis of case-control and cohort studies. *Vaccine*, *32*(29), 3623–3629.

Wilson, S. L., & Wiysonge, C. (2020). Social media and vaccine hesitancy. *BMJ Global Health*, *5*(10), e004206.

World Health Organization. (2019). Retrieved March 2019, from https://www.who.int/emergencies/ten-threats-to-global-health-in-2019

12

AUTHENTICITY AND MEDICAL COMMUNICATION SKILLS TRAINING

12.1 Introduction and rationale

How can Linguistics inform the way we train healthcare professionals to talk with patients?

Teaching and evaluating professional communication skills is complex, particularly in the globalized and intercultural contexts in which contemporary healthcare interactions occur. As touched on in Chapter 6, medical education, where the communication skills required for entry into the profession are taught to new practitioners, is an important site for linguistic research. It can tell us about the kinds of skills that become valued within medicine as well as how medical professionals become socially apprenticed into the field or, potentially, excluded.

This chapter showcases a study – Atkins (2019) 'Assessing health professionals' communication through role-play: An interactional analysis of simulated versus actual general practice consultations' – from medical education in the UK, addressing a licensing examination for General Practitioners (GP), in which the assessment of 'interpersonal skills' was a central component. The specific assessment, the Royal College of General Practitioners' Clinical Skills Assessment (CSA), was conducted through simulated consultations, where the GP performed role-played scenarios with actors playing the part of the patients. The exam came under scrutiny for its discrepant pass rates, particularly the much lower pass rates for international medical graduates (doctors who had taken their initial medical degree overseas but trained in the UK as general practitioners). The assessment of spoken communication skills was considered as one potential factor that might contribute to their poorer grading. Sociolinguists worked in conjunction with the Royal College of General Practitioners to look at linguistic and cultural factors that might be at play.

The broader study had many facets that have been reported on elsewhere (Roberts et al., 2014; Hawthorne et al., 2017) but one key area explored in this

DOI: 10.4324/9781003020417-15

chapter is the work by Atkins (2019) and Atkins et al. (2016), which looked par-ticularly at the effects of simulation on the interaction. 'Authenticity' was already touched on in Chapter 8 (see section 8.3.3). In this chapter, we address the idea of the 'authenticity' of simulated consultations compared to their real-life counterpart, using Corpus Linguistics and Conversation Analysis. The chapter provides ideas on comparative methods of analysis, including how one analytic step can inform the next and, in a data-driven approach, how it can point to further areas of explora-tion. The chapter also addresses how linguistic findings can be applied to real-life problems and the complexities of achieving 'impact' from healthcare research.

12.1.1 Key literature

Simulation and role-play are widely used in medical education, with tools such as 'Objective Structured Clinical Examinations' (OSCEs) designed to train and assess healthcare professionals' competencies through standardized, play-acted scenarios. Many studies have looked at whether simulations and role-play deliver an 'authentic' experience, with methods such as questionnaire studies used to establish whether participants find a simulation 'realistic' (Bosse et al., 2010). If designed well, it is argued that health professionals, 'cannot distinguish between real and well-trained simulated patients' (Kurtz et al., 1998: 62). However, the question of how far simulations can mimic the *talk* of real-life consultations was underexplored. This issue of the 'authenticity' of talk is important if we are considering the fairness and validity of such assessments for doctors preparing for real-life practice.

In thinking about authenticity in simulations, it is helpful to consider ideas around speakers' roles and identities, particularly 'asymmetry' in clinical con-texts (see Chapter 6, section 6.3.1). The asymmetry of the doctor–patient rela-tionship is a long-standing topic of discussion in medical sociology, with the doctor often conceptualized as an authoritative agent exerting power over the patient (Parsons, 1951). In this vein, simulations have sometimes been viewed as reversing this power asymmetry, 'because knowledge and judgement rest with the simulation patient rather than with the physician student' (Hanna & Fins, 2006: 266). As we discussed in Chapter 6, there is scope for power and expertise to be interactionally negotiated but it does seem hard to ignore the different interactional *contingencies* in simulation. Niements (2013) looks at role-plays of interpreter-mediated consultations, describing how they 'cannot reproduce the orientations of real interactions […] [W]hat is authentic to those users when they "live" a specific situation cannot be authentic to trainers/trainees when they play it' (Niements, 2013: 317). Outside the medical context, Stokoe (2011) too explores this phenomenon in professional role-play, suggesting the following:

> It is hard to support a claim that participants in role-play are oriented to the same interactional contingencies as they would be in the actual setting; even if participants rate role-playing as 'authentic' after the event […] For

those having their interactional skills evaluated, what is at stake is their performance and 'score' as trainees.

(Stokoe, 2011: 1653)

In seeking to understand authenticity and how participants negotiate these altered interactional contingencies in simulations, Atkins (2019) conducts a detailed, comparative analysis between simulated and real-life consultations, as set out below.

12.2 Methods and data

In addressing the authenticity of simulated CSA consultations, the specific questions this study aimed to answer were;

1. What key similarities and differences are there between the simulated exam cases and real general practice consultations?
2. Where there are differences, what might account for this within the design and contingencies of the role-played interaction?
3. Does the authenticity of the simulation matter for the assessment of healthcare professionals' communication skills?

Question 1 can be addressed through close analysis of spoken interaction: this involved collecting primary data from the CSA exam, taking place as part of the larger study on the exam outlined above, as well as drawing on a secondary, existing dataset of recorded GP consultations. The two datasets were then compared and analyzed using both corpus linguistic and conversation analytic (CA) approaches. Question 2 requires a broader, contextual consideration of the exam and its design, beyond just analysis of the spoken interaction itself, drawing on ethnographic field notes and discussions with examiners, GPs and other members of the Royal College of General Practitioners (see Chapters 2 and 6 on ethnography). Question 3 is not so much a matter for Linguistics as it is for medical education more broadly but points to the implications that these Linguistic findings had in the medical arena, which we discuss in section 12.4 below.

12.2.1 Data collection and practicalities

The data collection from the exam involved gaining consent from GP candidates to record their assessment and analyze this for research purposes. The process for this had to be agreed with a university research ethics committee beforehand, as outlined in Chapter 3. Ethically, the stress of the situation for the candidates, who were sitting an important professional examination, had to be carefully considered, making it clear that there was no obligation to take part and that it would have no bearing on their grading. In terms of mitigating any potential harm, a key consideration was in ensuring that those doctors who performed poorly in the assessment were not made identifiable. Successful candidates were asked for additional consent to use their videos as examples of good practice in training materials.

For this comparative study, a 'purposive sample', that is, a sample which covered the range of doctors' characteristics and backgrounds needed in the research, was taken from this cohort of 200 candidates, with equal numbers of passing and failing candidates, equal numbers of men and women as well as ethnic minority and international medical graduates. These 50 exam cases were transcribed in close detail using CLAN (see Chapter 6 on transcription), broadly following Jefferson (2004) conventions and indicating details such as overlapping talk, interruptions and pauses, yielding a dataset of 98,000 words.

In order to compare these simulated consultations, the researchers also needed a dataset of real-life GP consultations. For this, a corpus of consultations from GP surgeries in London was used, that had been collected for a previous project (Roberts et al., 2003). Though it would have been ideal to have a more contemporary corpus, this slightly older corpus of GP consultations was the one that the researchers had available. Collecting a new GP consultation dataset would have involved a further NHS ethics application, resourcing, and time that would not have been practical in the timescales for the project. Researchers often accept some limitations to the findings for a study, e.g. from using a slightly older dataset, in exchange for practicality. We also touch on the issue of 'imperfect' data in Chapter 10. The 'real' consultations dataset contained 37 consultations. This provided just over 110,000 words of interactional data, making it a roughly similar size to the exam dataset of 98,000 words above (though you will note here that the 37 real life consultations overall contained a greater number of words spoken than the 50 simulated ones).

12.2.2 Analytic methods

The comparison between these two specialist corpora was layered, involving both corpus linguistic and conversation analytic approaches. It began with a corpus overview of the data as a means of 'scoping out and quantifying recurring linguistic features' and enabling the identification of recurring patterns specific to the specialist context (Walsh, 2013: 45) (see also Chapters 7 and 8). Conversation Analysis (CA) of the transcripts, a qualitative, micro-analytic approach outlined in Chapter 6, formed the second layer of analysis, performing a closer investigation of the patterns that emerged from the quantitative analysis. The initial identification of patterns through corpus methods is one means of directing the researcher, from a data-driven position, to discourse segments that merit close analysis, with CA then providing a more granular understanding of the interactional sequences in which these features occur. In Atkins (2019), WordSmith Tools software (Scott, 2017) was used to identify recurrent single words and word clusters in each of the consultation datasets, and keyword comparisons were conducted between the two. Concordance lines were also examined for key phrases (3–5 word clusters), displaying the lexical items in their immediate linguistic context and enabling an initial analysis of the likely actions they perform (as in Example 12.1). From this initial corpus analysis, CA was then used to analyze how the phrases were employed in an interactional context, linking background information about the success or failure of candidates with endogenous evidence about the success of particular micro-interactional sequences.

12.3 Results and discussion

12.3.1 Corpus overview

The most frequent 3–5-word clusters were identified for both datasets and the results compared. From this corpus analysis, it was particularly notable that the most frequent word clusters in the simulated consultations (7 of the top 10), were all variants of the phrase, 'can you tell me a bit more about' / 'tell me a little bit more about' / 'tell me more about … ' and all spoken by the GP. These are referred to collectively in this study as 'tell me *more about' formulations. By contrast, Atkins (2019) highlights how this phrase did not occur at all in the top word clusters in the real-life GP consultations. Some phrases did show similarities across both datasets, such as various forms of the GP's initial elicitation request, 'how can I help'/'help you with today'/'what can I help', which occurred in the top 20 for both datasets. There were therefore some lexical parallels to suggest a degree of similarity between the two settings, real and simulated. Nevertheless, the difference with the 'tell me *more about' phrase was particularly stark and this was investigated through further qualitative analysis.

A plot of the 'tell me *more about' formulations showed the majority occurred at the start of the simulated consultations and a KWIC concordance output (Example 12.1) shows nearly all occurred as general requests by the GP candidate for further information:

EXAMPLE 12.1   Concordance of 'tell me a little/bit/more/about' cluster in the simulated consultations – sample of 20

N	Context (Left) **Keyword Cluster**	Context (Right)
1	oh you are ok can you **tell me a bit about**	that
2	all right ok (1.1) erm (1.1) t-t-**tell me about**	(0.3) you sister's baby (0.4)
3	un-huh ok can you **tell me a bit more**	about that
4	ok↘ yeah (0.8) ↑do you want to **tell me a bit more about**	it
5	cast a bit more (.) you know er **tell me a bit more about**	(.) why and how
6	ok **tell me a bit more about**	your symptoms *CASE NAME*
7	do you want to **tell me a bit more about**	it um (1.4)
8	(0.8) ok (0.7) um just um **tell me a bit more about**	what the reason why it was done
9	mmm can you **tell me a bit more about**	that
10	erm (.)can i ask (.)can can you **tell me a bit more about**	that (0.3)
11	(0.5) ok can you **tell me a bit more about**	that
12	right ok you want to **tell me a little bit about**	it
13	ok ·hhh um **tell me a little bit about**	what you know about vasectomy alrea
14	okay (0.8) do you want to **tell me a little bit more about**	it (0.6)
15	(1.9) can you **tell me a lit- little bit more**	(1.1)
16	(.) alright um (.) well **tell me a little bit more about**	your your periods and and how
17	coming today ok ·hhh do you want to **tell me a little bit more about**	it
18	why (0.5) **tell me a little bit more about**	(.)how long it's been going on
19	(0.5) ok (0.3) um (1.3) can you **tell me a lit- a little bit more about**	it (0.3) about your pe
20	you would be worried do you want to **tell me more about**	what happened on on on the on the day

By contrast, in the real GP consultations, the phrase occurred very infrequently (6 instances in all) and usually related to a much more specific request for information on a particular symptom, such as: 'just *tell me a bit more* they last fifteen twenty minutes you say'. Moreover, these types of requests occurred at a much later stage in the real GP consultations. Since this phrase occurred so consistently at the start of the simulated consultations, the decision was made to look across all the opening sequences of the 50 simulations, to analyze how it was used in interactional contexts.

12.3.2 Analysis of consultation openings

This section presents only a part of the CA analysis by Atkins (2019). Atkins chose to illustrate the findings using three opening excerpts from the *same* exam case performed by different candidate doctors – two of whom perform well and one who is unsuccessful in the case and exam overall. Limiting the initial excerpts to the same case allowed a more systematic presentation of the overall findings, perhaps avoiding the cherry-picking of cases from across the whole dataset.

The case is a complex one, involving a woman coming to the GP with the news that her sister's baby has been diagnosed with cystic fibrosis and seeking to enquire about inheritance risks. Under the criteria for the assessment, the candidate (CAN) must communicate the inheritance patterns for cystic fibrosis in an understandable manner, as well as demonstrate person-centred care and an understanding of the 'emotional impact' for the role-played patient (RPL). The following examples (Example 12.2 and Example 12.3) come from two successful candidates performing the opening few seconds of the consultation, and illustrate the general sequential patterns identified by Atkins (2019), culminating in the 'tell me *more about' phrase at lines 16 and line 20 respectively:

EXAMPLE 12.2   'Ms Ainscombe', Case 1 – PASS

```
1           ((BUZZER))
2    CAN: Joyce Ainscombe╱
3    RPL: yes≈
4    CAN: +≈ hello there╲
5    RPL: hi→
6    CAN: please have a seat my name is doctor Huang╱
7           (1.6)
8           ((EXM entering the room))
9    CAN: er: (.) how may I help you╲
10   RPL: ·hhhh my sister's baby has cystic fibrosis→
11   RPL: ·hhhh i was wondering whether my children would get this disease→
12   ges: [CAN nods]
13   CAN: mhm sorry to hear about your sister's╲
14   ges:                              [RPL nods]
15   CAN: erm (.) can I ask (.)
>16        can can you tell me a bit more about that
```

EXAMPLE 12.3 'Ms Ainscombe' Case 2 - PASS

```
    1           ((BUZZER))
    2             (0.4)
    3     CAN:  Joyce Ainscombe
    4     RPL:  hi
    5     CAN:  hi good morning please take a seat
    6     RPL:  hi
    7             (1.9)
    8     CAN:  my name is doctor Amari I'm one of the doctors here
    9           what can I do for you today
   10     RPL:  er my sister's baby has cystic fibrosis
   11             (0.7)
   12     RPL:  I was wondering whether
   13           my children will get this disease
   14     CAN:  oh dear (0.3) all right okay
   15           ·hhh
   16             (1.1)
   17     CAN:  ((CAN looks at notes))
   18           erm
   19             (0.9)
  >20     CAN:  t-t-tell me more about (0.3) you sister's⁄ baby⟍
```

After the initial opening buzzer and the 'hello/hi' greetings, we get several turns which have a similar sequential pattern across the simulated consultations, explored further below.

The simulations often began with an introduction designed as 'my name is doctor x' (Example 12.2, Line 6; Example 12.3, line 8), whereas the real consultations instead started with 'I'm doctor x'. This might seem an insignificant difference, but interestingly it aligned with the same finding about simulations versus real-life in a different professional setting – police interviews (Stokoe, 2013). Stokoe suggests this 'My name is … ' phrase may be a means of performing 'rapport-building' recommendations in the assessed simulation. The parallel to these GP consultations suggests this action may be a peculiarity of performing in simulated interactions.

Following the introduction, we get an initial inquiry (e.g. 'How can I help you' Example 12.2, line 9 and 'What can I do for you today' Example 12.3, line 9) and invite for the patient to speak. There are similar opening lines in real GP consultations, with the phrases found in both datasets in the corpus. We then see the role-players deliver the scripted opening lines for the case, giving a two-part account and enquiry in each: 'my sister's baby has cystic fibrosis – I was wondering whether my children would get this disease' (Example 12.2, line 10–11 and Example 12.3, line 10). In each we have some acknowledgement or 'receipt token' from the candidate indicating the distressing nature of the news ('sorry to hear'; 'oh dear'). Both candidates follow up the receipt or empathy token with a 'tell me *more about' request for further information (Example 12.2, line 15–16, Example 12.3, line 20), the frequent word-cluster identified by the corpus analysis. This action was performed in a very consistent sequential position across the 50 simulated cases. It is worth noting that, although this question is designed to get some more information from the patient role-player, it did not usually result in a very long response, meaning that the doctor had to continue asking further questions to gain information about the patient's background.

In the real consultations, Atkins (2019) does not find this phrase or sequence to be present in the opening moments. Instead, the opening query from the doctor, such as 'how can I help you today' was shown to elicit a much longer response from the patient, giving a narrative outline of their symptoms. There was no need for the GP to follow up with a 'tell me *more about … ' formulation because the patient usually volunteered a wealth of information themselves. In one case from the real-life consultations, after the opening enquiry, the patient holds the floor for the first 5 minutes and 32 seconds before the doctor comes in with a more structured set of questions. Although not all cases are so extreme, research on general practice has shown that patients who know the format of the consultation produce an almost pre-prepared narrative at the outset of the inter-action (McKinley & Middleton, 1999).

From the corpus linguistic and CA analyses, there appeared to be a convention-alized sequence built up in the simulations that did not mimic real-life and that, when not followed correctly, could lead to considerable difficulties for less suc-cessful doctors in the exam. Difficulties seemed to occur when opportunities for delivering empathy phrases were missed and when formulaic questions (such as 'tell me *more about') were delivered on the wrong topic or at the wrong interactional juncture (i.e. not in the conventional sequences shown above). In real-life GP con-sultations, there also appeared to be greater scope for repair than in the simulated exam setting, where the participation framework can shift to afford greater power to the role-player, and for the candidate to be put on the back foot.

These findings suggest ways in which role-play and simulation might not always be a fair means of assessing communication skills for healthcare profes-sionals, testing different competencies to real-life practice and benefiting those with tacit knowledge of the interactional patterns of role-play. This may be a par-ticular difficulty for overseas doctors: OSCEs and simulation for assessing inter-personal skills are not always employed to the same extent across Undergraduate medical curricula internationally and the conventionalized communication needed to perform well may be difficult to acculturate to, particularly since the training GPs' experience prior to the exam takes place in largely real-life clinical practice settings.

12.4 Impact

'Impact' is a term used to describe the beneficial effects that research can have on society and the economy, beyond academia (cf. REF, 2021 guidelines). This involves more than just reporting 'findings' from research and can happen in various ways, such as changes to policy, reframing key debates and shifts in eve-ryday practice. Research projects on interaction in healthcare settings often have real potential to feed into policy and practice, although the routes to achieving this can take work, usually requiring researchers to engage with non-language specialists and find audiences and outlets beyond their disciplinary field.

The impact of this research project was twofold: changing training for GPs and reframing the debate around discrepant pass rates. Firstly, then, findings about the communicative competencies needed for performing well in the simulated consultations of the assessment were fed into evidence-based training materials for GPs who were preparing for the exam. Some scholars, such as Seale et al. (2007) have commented that simulated medical consultations might be more interactionally demanding than their real-life counterpart – the close linguistic analysis by Atkins (2019) goes some way to showing what those increased demands might be, all of which may be useful to GPs preparing for the assessment. The educational materials presented findings from the analysis and were delivered through e-learning modules, a textbook (Rolfe et al., 2015) and face-to-face workshops for GPs (detailed further in Atkins, 2022).

However, it was also important to the researchers that training outputs not be the only impact of the work, with the concern that the research should not simply reinforce a 'deficit model' for GP trainees who performed more poorly in the assessment. As further impact, the researchers wanted to ensure that more critical findings about the problems with using simulation for assessing real-life competencies fed into policies and changes around the exam. This more controversial impact was a much trickier outcome to achieve and required ongoing meetings and involvement with the RCGP (detailed in Atkins, 2022, and Roberts, 2021). Some changes were achieved in the way the interpersonal skills domain was assessed, but much of this impact involved subtler, longer-term shifts in the way the College used terminology and made changes to the exam over the course of years – arguably more far-reaching impact but much harder to measure than workshops and training materials.

12.5 Conclusions

Linguistic methods and frameworks offered a useful means of comparing datasets in this study. Corpus linguistic methods were employed as an initial exploratory approach to direct the focus for the subsequent Conversation Analysis. Both methods have been covered in this book and could be similarly applied to other settings. In making such comparisons, linguists rarely have perfectly equivalent datasets and some limitations may have to be accepted, such as a difference in time period covered by the two sets of transcripts. Nevertheless, these approaches offer a way into understanding real-life questions around 'authenticity' and fairness in the assessment of communication skills that other fields cannot, showing the real value and potential for impact from linguistic research in healthcare.

References

Atkins, S. (2019). Assessing health professionals' communication through role-play: An interactional analysis of simulated versus actual general practice consultations. *Discourse Studies, 21*(2), 109–134.

Atkins, S. (2022). The ethics of engagement: Research relationships in an applied linguistics partnership with a professional medical body. *Journal of Applied Linguistics and Professional Practice, 17*(1), 1–23.

Atkins, S., Roberts, C., Hawthorne, K., & Greenhalgh, T. (2016). Simulated consultations: A sociolinguistic perspective. *BMC Medical Education, 16*(16), 1–9. https://doi.org/10 .1186/s12909-016-0535-2, PMID: 26768421; PMCID: PMC4714536.

Bosse, H. M., Nickel, M., Huwendiek, S., Jünger, J., Schultz, J. H., & Nikendei, C. (2010). Peer role-play and standardised patients in communication training: A comparative study on the student perspective on acceptability, realism, and perceived effect. *BMC Medical Education, 10*(27), 1–9. https://bmcmededuc.biomedcentral.com /articles/10.1186/1472-6920-10-27.

Hanna, M., & Fins, J. (2006) Power and communication: Why simulation training ought to be complemented by experiential and humanist learning. *Academic Medicine, 81*(3), 265–270.

Hawthorne, K., Roberts, C., & Atkins, S. (2017). Sociolinguistic factors affecting performance in the clinical skills assessment of the MRCGP: A mixed-methods approach. *British Journal of General Practice (Open), 1*(1), 1–9.

Jefferson, G. (2004). Glossary of transcript symbols with an introduction. In G. Lerner (Ed.), *Conversation analysis: Studies from the first generation* (pp. 13–31). John Benjamins.

Kurtz, S., Silverman, J., & Draper, J. (1998). *Teaching and learning communication skills in medicine.* Radcliffe Medical Press.

McKinley, R., & Middleton, J. (1999). What do patients want from doctors? Content analysis of written patient agendas for the consultation. *British Journal of General Practice, 49*(447), 796–800.

Niemants, N. (2013). From role-playing to role-taking: Interpreter's role(s) in healthcare. In C. Schäffner, K. Kredens & Y. Fowler (Eds.), *Interpreting in a changing landscape: Selected papers from critical link* (pp. 305–319). John Benjamins.

Parsons, T. (1951). *The social system.* Free Press.

Research Excellence Framework (REF). (2021). *Guide to the REF results.* Retrieved from https://rcf.ac.uk/guidance-on-results/guidance-on-ref-2021-results/#:~:text =For%20REF%202021%2C%20impact%20is,quality%20of%20life%2C%20beyond %20academia

Roberts, C. (2021). *Linguistic penalties and the job interview.* Equniox.

Roberts, C., Atkins, S., & Hawthorne, K. (2014). *Performance features in clinical skills assessment: Linguistic and cultural factors in the membership of the Royal College of General Practitioners examination.* King's College London; University of Nottingham.

Roberts, C., Moss, B., Wass, V., Sarangi, S., & Jones, R. (2003). *The PLEDGE project (Patients with Limited English and Doctors in General Practice).* King's College London.

Rolfe, A., Atkins, S., Hawthorne, K., & Roberts, C. (2015). *The insider's guide to the clinical skills assessment for the MRCGP.* Royal College of General Practitioners.

Scott, M. (2017). *Wordsmith tools version 7.* Lexical Analysis Software.

Seale, C., Butler, C., Hutchby, I., Kinnersley, P., & Rollnick, S. (2007). Negotiating frame ambiguity: A study of simulated encounters in medical education. *Communication and Medicine, 4*(2), 177–187.

Stokoe, E. (2011). Simulated interaction and communication skills training: The 'conversation analytic role-play method'. In C. Antaki (Ed.), *Applied conversation analysis: Changing institutional practices* (pp. 119–139). Palgrave Macmillan.

Stokoe, E. (2013). The (In)authenticity of simulated talk: Comparing role-played and actual interaction and the implications for communication training. *Research on Language and Social Interaction*, *46*(2), 165–185. https://doi.org/10.1080/08351813.2013.780341.

Walsh, S. (2013). Corpus linguistics and conversation analysis at the interface: Theoretical perspectives, practical outcomes. In J. Romero-Trillo (Ed.), *Yearbook of corpus linguistics and pragmatics 2013: New domains and methodologies* (pp. 37–51). Springer.

13

STORYTELLING AND AFFILIATION AMONGST HEALTHCARE PROFESSIONALS

13.1 Introduction and rationale

Strains on healthcare staff, who often work long hours in stressful and some-times upsetting environments, have become well recognized, especially fol-lowing the Covid-19 pandemic. This can make the task of caring for patients all the more challenging, with staff described as suffering from 'compassion fatigue' and 'burn out'. How can healthcare organizations recognize and sup-port staff in roles where emotionally difficult situations arise? It is well-known that, more than simply exchanging information, communication can be a key means for building relationships, identities, and for fostering a sense of community between people. One interesting context for inter-professional communication between healthcare staff established in more recent years, particularly in the US, Canada, UK, and Australia and New Zealand, are 'Schwartz Center Rounds'. Schwartz Rounds are supportive, interdisciplinary forums designed for healthcare staff to talk to each other in informal ways, enabling people to reflect on emotional, ethical, and social complexities of their jobs when caring for patients. Here we showcase the study 'Storytelling and affiliation between groups of healthcare staff in Schwartz Round inter-actions' (Atkins et al., forthcoming) on how interactional storytelling is employed in Schwartz Rounds in the UK to help foster a sense of support and wellbeing among hospital staff.

Given the sensitive nature of the setting, this was a difficult site to gain access to. While you may not be collecting such complex data in your own research, we wanted to include this case study to demonstrate the value as well as flag some complexities of looking at health interactions other than those involving patients (see Chapter 6). Looking at this type of inter-professional talk highlights how issues of wellbeing affect staff in healthcare too and how this area overlaps

DOI: 10.4324/9781003020417-16

with linguistic research on organizational communication. Most importantly, the case study provides a practical overview of how complex ethical issues for collecting and analyzing sensitive data can be addressed during a relatively short 1-year research project, building on guidance given in Chapter 3. These are strategies you may be able to draw on if you are preparing an ethics application for your own project, particularly if you are approaching sensitive topics with your participants.

Schwartz Rounds originally started in the US, with Ken Schwartz founding the 'Schwartz Center' in 1995. His vision was for an organization that would foster compassionate care from healthcare staff, recognizing from his own experiences the 'acts of kindness – the simple human touch from my caregivers' that, 'have made the unbearable bearable' (www.theschwartzcenter.org /about/who-we-are/). Schwartz Rounds were introduced to the UK in 2009 through the *Point of Care Foundation*, and are now run at over 220 UK hospital trusts and healthcare organizations. In the UK, each Schwartz Round follows roughly the same structure, lasting an hour and beginning with an introduction by a 'clinical lead' or a 'facilitator', followed by a multidisciplinary panel of 3–4 members of staff, presenting stories of personal experience to an audience of other staff members from across the organization. These stories are prepared in advance, with the Round facilitator meeting with panellists and guiding them in how to craft their story. After panellists have delivered their stories in the Round, the facilitator then guides the follow up discussion, allowing audiences to reflect on similar experiences and themes. The principle is that these forums should give staff time and space to reflect on and talk about experiences in their job, with the rationale that this, in turn, will help staff with the task of caring for patients.

It is easy to see some links here to Narrative Medicine and the Medical Humanities mentioned in Chapters 5 and 8. Indeed, Charon (2006) references the work of the Schwartz Center in the US in describing possible training for professionals. Storytelling in this setting could therefore be addressed through a number approaches outlined in this book. In Atkins et al. (forthcoming), the researchers draw on an evaluation by Maben et al. (2018) and use Conversation Analysis (see Chapter 6), to explore how storytelling and affiliation are performed between hospital staff interacting in Rounds. The ways in which staff communicate to show their affiliation and create a sense of support is helpful to explore using linguistic methods: the setting is conspicuously aimed at nurturing staff wellbeing and compassionate care, with the facility to tell stories and share experiences through talk seen as a central function. The space to share experiences has been identified as a mechanism through in which Rounds actually work, with Maben et al. (2018) highlighting how this triggers reflection and resonance with others' experiences (p. 108). It seems reasonable to claim, given the particular nature of the setting, that the interactional features of Schwartz Rounds are important to their successful function in establishing supportive relationships amongst staff.

13.1.1 Key literature

Storytelling and listeners' responses have been well-noted in conversation analytic work (e.g. Sacks, 1986, Stivers, 2008). In telling stories, speakers do not just recount events that have happened but also convey their 'affective treatment of the events' or their *stance* toward them, indicating the kind of responses they might expect from recipients (Stivers, 2008: 27). Stivers (2008) defined two concepts in how recipients respond to storytellers: *alignment* (defined as a 'structural level of cooperation' with the activity) and *affiliation* (an 'affective level of cooperation'). Aligned responses are those which cooperate with the storytelling activity, such as providing short continuers ('mhm') during a speaker's story to allow them to continue (Stivers et al., 2011: 20). Affiliative responses, though, associate the recipient with the *stance* conveyed by the storyteller, often showing empathy or agreement (Stivers et al., 2011: 21). There is a preference to display this affiliation, particularly where a speaker recounts a story with some degree of emotional intensity, which Heritage (2011) suggests creates 'empathic moments' in the talk. Drawing on this prior research, we turn to storytelling and affiliation in the Rounds.

13.2 Methods and data

The research questions for this study were:

1. How is storytelling performed by hospital staff in Schwartz Rounds?
2. How is 'affiliation' (and sometimes disaffiliation) interactionally achieved in participants' responses to stories?
3. Which communicative features contribute to a sense of shared experience and support in Schwartz Rounds?

Questions 1 and 2 aim to describe in detail the communication that takes place in Schwartz Rounds and require the collection of naturally occurring data from Rounds, described in the next section. In addressing Question 3, the researchers drew on interview and focus group data from Maben et al.'s (2018) realist-informed review to broaden the scope in thinking about what is achieved through these kinds of communicative events. Even where researchers do not have the kind of rich ethnographic involvement with research sites outlined in Chapter 6, they can still draw on existing secondary data and literature to bring an understanding of the context to their analysis. Similarly to Chapter 10, where Semino drew on the findings of existing research and data to analyze Covid-19 metaphors, research questions can be answered in different ways and with different sources of evidence.

13.2.1 Data collection and ethical considerations

The primary data collection for this study involved recording five full-length (1-hour) Schwartz Rounds across 3 hospitals in the UK. Schwartz Rounds are clearly a sensitive setting and staff are asked to keep people's contributions anonymous so that everyone can feel safe and secure in speaking. Recording these settings for research, whether through audio or video, ran the risk of breaking that trust and safety, with the potential to cause social and relational damage, as we discussed in Chapter 3. Though the adults involved in the Schwartz Rounds would not typically be described as 'vulnerable' and all had capacity to give consent for such recordings, the Schwartz Round setting is, by its nature, one in which people frequently present emotionally difficult issues in relation to their work, so that participants can become vulnerable through the distressing nature of the activity.

A major consideration in thinking about how to collect data was therefore around how to record and analyse interactions respectfully, without causing undue distress to participants. Data collection was made more complex through the fact that Schwartz Rounds can be very large events (across an entire hospital) and there is no requirement for staff to pre-book their attendance. In the era before Covid-19, when this study was conducted, they could simply 'drop in' to a lunchtime Round, meaning that gaining consent from all participants, in the days and weeks prior to the event, would have been impractical. It needed to be conducted by researchers on site, at the event itself.

Previous Schwartz Rounds had in fact been filmed for training and promotion purposes and so Atkins et al. built on the precedent for this to establish an ethics procedure, with input from Schwartz Round steering groups at a number of hospitals as to what they felt would be practical. The Schwartz Round framework already considered the emotionally complex issues that might arise from Rounds discussions, particularly in the support provided to panellists before and after sessions. The researchers therefore sought to support this existing process, planning to closely consult with the facilitators for each Round beforehand as to what they felt would be the likely ethical challenges.

Once the processes and practicalities had been discussed with steering groups, the researchers set out a 5-step ethics protocol and applied for ethical approval. Example 13.1 gives the revised and agreed plan, as it appeared in the final ethics application:

EXAMPLE 13.1   Excerpt from the ethics application for the Schwartz Round project

What arrangements are to be made to obtain the free and informed consent of the participants?

The 5-step procedure to be followed for both audio and video recordings, will be:

1. **Discuss and agree recordings with SR steering group at a hospital trust or other organisation.**
   Organisations that run Schwartz Rounds will be approached via an introduction through the Point of Care Foundation, who oversee the conduct of Rounds in the UK.

2. **Consent to record a Round is discussed well in advance with facilitators and the planned panellists.**

    The clinical lead, facilitator and steering group will be approached in scoping out the possibility for conducting a recorded Round, according to the ethical principles set out here. The clinical lead and the facilitator (who are to appear in the recording) will have autonomy over the decision to record and will of course have the opportunity to ask the research team questions prior to making a decision.

    Subsequently, panellists who suggest they are happy to be recorded for a Round will have the opportunity to discuss the research and prepare their story in advance with the facilitator (having the option to withdraw from the research at this stage if they prefer). The clinical lead, facilitator and panellists will all therefore be consented well in advance of the Round.

3. **Intention to record the Round clearly communicated beforehand – posters and all communications prior to the Round (researcher contact details provided). The information sheet will be shared in communications prior to the Round.**

    Audience members for Rounds are difficult to predict in advance (it is entirely voluntary to attend a Schwartz Round on the day). We will therefore follow the procedures of previous organisations in recording Rounds. The Schwartz Round team will indicate in communications well in advance of the Round of the intention to record (through posters, emails etc.), so that this does not come as a surprise to audience members on the day. Contact details of the research fellow (Sarah Atkins) will be provided in order to answer any questions prior to the event.

4. **Audience members will receive a hard copy of the information sheet and consent form for recording at the check in desk on the day. The lunch period that takes place before a Round will be used to give participants time to consider the information and whether to participate – and they can leave at this point if they choose. For video recorded Rounds, audience members can request to be seated outside of the sight of cameras if they choose.**

    Current procedures mean that all participants in Rounds must sign in at a reception desk on arrival, so, as with previous Rounds, an extra step of consenting to the recording will be put in place for each participant at the sign-in desk.

5. **After the event, audience members, panellists, facilitators or members of the steering group can request that any section of the recording be deleted or anonymised. The researcher will check with the facilitator, following the panel debrief, if any issues were raised with the recording**.

    Following the recording, any member of the audience can request to have their section of the recording either fully removed or anonymised (through pixilation) and may request this for up to one month after the event (date to be provided on the information sheet and consent form). Similarly, the panellists, clinical lead and facilitator are able to discuss, following the session, whether sections of the recording should be deleted or anonymised (through pixilation).

The ethics application also indicated that researchers should consider the risks of participants disclosing 'issues of concern' – that is, potentially 'reportable disclosures' where a participant gives information that indicates a risk to people's safety or wellbeing that must be reported in order that it can be prevented. This question is not unusual in ethics applications and is something you may need to consider with data-collection methods such as interviews. Here, however, this highlights the complexities of conducting research with external organizations, since this risk of reportable disclosures was one already addressed by the Point of Care Foundation and hospital trusts. The Point of Care Foundation trained facilitators in dealing with these instances (though it should be noted they occur very infrequently) and the researchers had to emphasize in the ethics application that they must work within the protocols of the organization, should these kinds of disclosures occur.

Finally, as well as these risks to participants, the ethics application also acknowledged some risks to the researchers, a topic discussed in Chapter 3 (see section 3.5). This was the outline written at the time of application in 2019:

> There are no physical safety risks to the researcher, since all Schwartz Rounds take place in public forums (in hospitals and other professional settings), which have already been risk assessed for use, including for external visitors. However, Schwartz Rounds often discuss emotionally complex situations which can be upsetting for researchers to transcribe and analyse. It has been suggested that researcher safety (including psychological safety) should be a central methodological concern (Mitchell & Irvine, 2008; Hughes, 2004). The research team will seek to support all staff (including transcribers) in the manner recommended for this type of research (see Fahie, 2014) – through highlighting the emotionally complex nature of the content, maintaining regular discussion with the team and allowing time for debrief sessions with the project PI and Director of the Centre.

Since 2019, there has been considerably more attention given to the risks of working with distressing data, with a new section added to the BAAL *Recommendations for Good Practice in Applied Linguistics* (BAAL, 2021). Thinking about the same project a few years down the line, it would be appropriate to elaborate further on the plans above by including the potential to access more formal psychological support, as well as good practices for working with such data, such as allocating set times for transcription and analysis.

The process of gaining approval was not entirely straightforward and the researchers had to field several queries and suggestions from the university ethics committee about changing the research protocols, some of which the researchers took on board, particularly in the practicalities of consenting a large number of people at the Round check-in desks. However, one suggestion made was that it may be more ethical to simulate the interactions, rather than record the 'real thing', given the potentially distressing nature of the setting for participants. Since a central tenet of Discourse and Conversation Analysis is to work with naturally occurring data, and the project aimed to produce evidence-based materials for facilitators, the researchers rejected this suggestion. They explained to the ethics committee why it would have been methodologically difficult, particularly given the established differences between real interactions and their simulated counterparts (see Chapter 12). This response was ultimately received favourably by the ethics committee and a final consent process agreed.

Overall, gaining approval took five months. Fielding discussions between hospital steering groups and the university ethics committee inevitably made this a lengthy process. Many projects engaged with external organizations face challenges of meeting the requirements of different parties. A five month timeframe was particularly tricky for a project that had funding for only a year. However, it should also be emphasized that this was also not wasted time – in establishing these procedures, the researcher built strong relationships with the healthcare trusts and had time to visit, participate, and gain an ethnographic understanding of the settings (see section 6.3.3). Building these relationships also aided a smooth data-collection process once approval was gained.

13.2.2 Methods

Transcripts using Jefferson's (2004) conventions were made for each 1-hour Round, a notation system described in Chapter 6 which captures the compositional qualities (choice of vocabulary, prosody, speed) and sequential order of the talk. Names of people and locations were anonymized, with pseudonyms used in the transcripts (see Chapter 3. section 3.4 on anonymizing data). Conversation Analysis (CA), as a qualitative, micro-analytic approach to talk outlined in Chapter 6, was appropriate to apply to this dataset, particularly with the interest in storytelling and the interactional opportunities for affiliation to be expressed (c.f. Sacks, 1986; Stivers, 2008; Stivers et al., 2011; Heritage, 2011). This provided prior research and terminology to draw on, including 'second stories', and 'endorsements', terms outlined further below.

13.3 Results and discussion

In answering research questions 1 and 2, the bulk of the study addressed the micro-interactional processes through which stories are performed and affiliation is expressed by the audience.

13.3.1 Storytelling

In Schwartz Rounds, the storytellers on the panel are explicitly given the right to the floor (e.g., in the example below, the clinical lead hands over the floor to the panellist, 'so Luke over to you please', line 105). This means panellists do not have to 'project' their upcoming story (i.e. communicate their intention to listeners that they intend to tell a story and wish to hold the floor for an extended period) in the same way as in casual conversation, since turn-taking rights are expressly suspended. Nevertheless, panellists still sometimes gave a short preface about the ensuing story listeners could expect, before launching into their narratives:

EXAMPLE 13.2   Extract from Round 1

```
105      LEAD: Tk- thank you very much so *Luke* (0.2) over to you (.) please.
106      PAUS: (0.4)
107   →  PAN1: So I'm just going t- give a little bit as those that have been
108   →        before will know of of um this case.
109            so this was a little girl called *Cara* (0.5) e:rm who
110            wa:s born just a little early...
```
(Round 1, lines 105-113)

This panellist's story preface explicitly positions his action of giving 'a very brief outline' (line 108, Example 13.2) as being appropriate to the Schwartz Round context ('as those of you that have been before will know' line 107-8), positioning himself as an experienced speaker who knows the conventions of this setting. The panellist then goes on to give an account of the difficult experience of advising the family that their newborn baby will not survive. Following this panellist's account, two further, interconnected stories are given from other members of the same medical team, a feature that was common in 'case-based' rounds, where the same patient case is described by different members of staff.

13.3.2 Endorsements

Many audience members provided a positive evaluation of the stories and the emotions expressed in Rounds, showing affiliation in the sense Stivers (2008: 35) describes; 'the hearer displays support of and endorses the teller's conveyed stance'. Interestingly, though, the researchers also found that these endorsements could be more 'metapragmatic' in nature, a term drawn from Linguistics (cf. Verschueren, 2022), rather than CA. By this they meant that, rather than always endorsing the emotions or attitudes the panellists expressed, instead the audience members would often endorse the *act* of expressing those difficult experiences and emotions at all (e.g. 'thank you for sharing that'). This is a potentially important function in a support-group setting, where difficult and sometimes controversial emotions are being expressed (such as frustration with patients).

13.3.3 Second stories

In CA, second stories are narratives given in response to another speaker's story, designed to show they are touched off by or pick up on the point of the first story (Sacks, 1992, Goodwin, 1990; Gardner, 1971). A stated aim of Schwartz

Rounds, and an aim you can see expressed by facilitators, is to inspire stories of similar experiences from the audience (e.g. '… now is your opportunity for to-to- actually reflect for yourself on some of those (0.5) erm moments that maybe you've had something happening that was similar … '). Sometimes, second stories in the recorded Rounds did give an account describing a similar difficulty. For example, Example 13.3 gives the opening to one such second story:

EXAMPLE 13.3   Second story in a Schwartz Round

```
654  AUD3:  I just wanted to >talk about< it's nothing gra:nd
655         compared to what you guys are doing=but I had a
656         (.) .h >I< I treat a patient () patient er with
657         with polycystic kidney disease (0.7) and…
```

(Round 4, lines 654-657)

It is interesting that the speaker, at the opening to her second story here, stops herself after 'I just wanted to >talk about<' and, as a politeness strategy, adds a quick interjection that downplays how comparable her experiences are – 'it's nothing grand compared to what you guys are doing', before then giving an account of a patient she is treating with kidney disease. She goes on to provide an account of a change she is proud to have achieved, mirroring panellists' stories about achieving change and overcoming obstacles. Second stories recounting similar experiences are relatively common in Rounds, but there was often a hesitancy or sensitivity expressed by speakers in claiming equivalence in experience. This difficulty in claiming identical experiences to others' very 'exceptional' stories has been noted in help group settings such as AA meetings (Arminen, 2004) and was something that contributors expressed in their responses in this setting.

13.3.4 *Shared experience and support in Schwartz Rounds*

In looking at the details of the talk in Schwartz Rounds, Atkins et al. (forthcoming) are able to set out some features that may actually achieve the social effects found to be beneficial to staff. Maben et al. (2018) found that participants commented on the value of the group connections enabled through giving and responding to shared experiences:

> it's kind of 'oh I didn't know it was like that for you'. I think it strengthens the connections and the relationships with other people (…)

In particular, the ways in which audience members respond to panellists' initial stories can be a means through which a sense of affiliation and joint experience is achieved. The importance of gaining these responses in Rounds can be seen in some of the interview data collected by Maben et al. (2018), particularly where their absence is noted:

Actually nobody responded to my story at all [...] And I actually found that quite difficult 'cause I couldn't work out why that was and I felt like I'd actually made myself really quite vulnerable there [...] and so I felt like I probably overstretched myself in terms of thinking it would be all right to present her and maybe it wasn't [...] and because I then didn't – people didn't respond to me, I didn't know why that was, and maybe it was too difficult for other people, as well [...] I kind of regretted doing it afterwards.

(Elderberry-2-Facilitator-speaking-as-Panellist)

For this Schwartz Round panellist, simply having space to recount a story was not sufficient for the Round to feel like a helpful experience – there needed to be responses from the audience that expressed an understanding of the themes and emotional stance articulated, i.e. for this to be an *affiliative* interaction. This is akin to conversation analytic findings, where recipients are expected to give the types responses outlined above (Mandelbaum, 2013: 505). Such findings have implications for Round facilitators in the tricky task of guiding discussions and ensuring the audience can find ways to respond to what are accounts of often very exceptional experiences.

13.4 Conclusions

The study we have discussed builds on a well-known body of literature about interactional storytelling and affiliation. In using these methods to identify interactional features that achieve affiliation in Schwartz Rounds, some practical insights for facilitators wishing to aid discussion in these settings can be provided. It also gives insight into the ways healthcare practitioners and staff from across different settings are able to find commonalities in their experiences and achieve some sense of shared identity through talk.

Research in this sensitive context involved considerable challenges for data collection, set out in detail above. Ethically this meant considering the best ways to respect and protect participants when collecting data from what are usually private events. In terms of more procedural aspects, this involved fielding discussions with both the research sites and the university ethics committee to establish a consent process that would be both considerate of and practical for a large number of participants to complete. These kinds of difficulties require planning for a larger project, particularly where there are strict time-bound limitations.

References

Arminen, I. (2004). Second stories: The salience of interpersonal communication for mutual help in alcoholics anonymous. *Journal of Pragmatics, 36*(2), 319–347.

Atkins, S., Pilnick, A., Maben, J., & Thompson, L. (forthcoming). Storytelling and affiliation between groups of healthcare staff in Schwartz Round interactions: a conversation analytic study.

British Association for Applied Linguistics (BAAL). (2021). *Recommendations on good practice in applied linguistics.* Retrieved from https://www.baal.org.uk/wp-content/uploads/2021/03/BAAL-Good-Practice-Guidelines-2021.pdf

Charon, R. (2006). *Narrative medicine: Honoring the stories of illness.* Oxford University Press.

Fahie, D. (2014). Doing sensitive research sensitively: Ethical and methodological issues in researching workplace bullying. *International Journal of Qualitative Methods, 13*(1), 19–36.

Gardner, R. A. (1971). *Therapeutic communication with children: The mutual storytelling technique.* Jason Aronson.

Goodwin, M. H. (1990). *He-said-she-said: Talk as social organization among black children.* Indiana University Press.

Heritage, J. (2011). Territories of knowledge, territories of experience: Empathic moments in interaction. In T. Stivers, L. Mondada, & J. Steensig (Eds.), *The morality of knowledge in conversation* (pp. 159–183). Cambridge University Press.

Hughes, R. (2004). Safety in nursing social research. *International Journal of Nursing Studies, 41*(8), 933–940.

Jefferson, G. (2004). Glossary of transcript symbols with an introduction. In G. H. Lerner (Ed.), *Conversation analysis: Studies from the first generation* (pp. 13–34). John Benjamins.

Maben, J., Taylor, C., Dawson, J., Leamy, M., McCarthy, I., Reynolds, E., Ross, S., Shuldham, C., Bennett, L., & Foot, C. (2018). A realist informed mixed-methods evaluation of Schwartz Center Rounds® in England. *Health Services and Delivery Research, 6*(37). Retrieved from https://www.ncbi.nlm.nih.gov/books/NBK533086/

Mandelbaum, J. (2013). Storytelling in conversation. In J. Sidnell & T. Stivers (Eds.), *The handbook of conversation analysis* (pp. 492–507). John Wiley & Sons.

Mitchell, W., & Irvine, A. (2008). I'm okay, you're okay?: Reflections on the well-being and ethical requirements of researchers and research participants in conducting qualitative fieldwork interviews. *International Journal of Qualitative Methods, 7*(4), 31–44.

Sacks, H. (1986). Some considerations of a story told in ordinary conversation. *Poetics, 15*(1–2), 127–138.

Sacks, H. (1992). *Lectures on conversation (Vols 1 & 2).* Blackwell.

Stivers, T. (2008). Stance, alignment, and affiliation during storytelling: When nodding is a token of affiliation. *Research on Language and Social Interaction, 41*(1), 31–57.

Stivers, T., Mondada, L., & Steensig, J. (2011). Knowledge, morality and affiliation in social interaction. In *The morality of knowledge in conversation* (pp. 3–24). Cambridge University Press.

Verschueren, J. (2022). Metapragmatics. In J.-O. Östman & J. Verschueren (Eds.), *Handbook of pragmatics: Manual* (2nd ed.), (pp. 948–953). John Benjamins.

INDEX